Clinical Oral Medicine and Pathology

Jean M. Bruch • Nathaniel S. Treister

Clinical Oral Medicine and Pathology

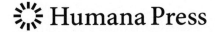 Humana Press

Jean M. Bruch, DMD, MD
Massachusetts Eye and Ear Infirmary
Boston, MA
jean_bruch@meei.harvard.edu

Nathaniel S. Treister, DMD
Brigham and Women's Hospital
Boston, MA
ntreister@partners.org

ISBN 978-1-60327-519-4   e-ISBN 978-1-60327-520-0
DOI 10.1007/978-1-60327-520-0
Springer New York Dordrecht Heidelberg London

Library of Congress Control Number: 2009927497

Springer is part of Springer Science+Business Media (www.springer.com)

Preface

What is *oral medicine*? Broadly speaking, it is the field of medicine that encompasses the diagnosis and management of diseases affecting the oral cavity. Many conditions produce oral signs and symptoms, and yet the oral cavity is an unfamiliar zone for many clinicians. Physicians generally receive little formal training in dental and oral medicine, and tend to view the oral cavity as a place reserved for their "dental" colleagues. Likewise, dentists are experts in the diagnosis and management of diseases related to the teeth and periodontium; however, the proportion of dental education dedicated to the "non-dental" part of the oral cavity often falls short. For these reasons, it is not at all uncommon for a patient to visit five to ten doctors before receiving a correct diagnosis and appropriate treatment plan, often months to years following onset of symptoms. It was from this landscape that this book was designed and written.

Given the wide range of clinical presentations, patients with oral complaints may seek out or be referred to a variety of health care providers, including primary care physicians, dentists, otolaryngologists, oral surgeons, dermatologists, neurologists, psychiatrists, and rheumatologists. Many of these oral conditions can be recognized and managed without the need for additional specialty referral. In this book, we have attempted to provide a rational, concise, and yet comprehensive approach to the practice of oral medicine for all those who are likely to encounter diseases of the oral cavity in their daily practice. We have included specific guidelines on diagnosis, management, and follow-up. Our intent was to create a clinically relevant and accessible resource for health care professionals, truly bridging the worlds of dentistry and medicine.

About the Authors

Jean M. Bruch, DMD, MD

Dr. Bruch earned her DMD from Harvard School of Dental Medicine in 1989 and MD from Harvard Medical School in 1991. She subsequently completed surgical residency training programs in oral and maxillofacial surgery at Massachusetts General Hospital and otolaryngology at Massachusetts Eye and Ear Infirmary as well as a fellowship in laryngology. She practices otolaryngology at Massachusetts Eye and Ear Infirmary with special interest in laryngology, thyroid surgery, and oral diseases. She is an instructor in laryngology and otology at Harvard Medical School and spends time teaching medical students and otolaryngology residents.

Nathaniel S. Treister, DMD, DMSc

Dr. Treister earned his DMD from the University of Pennsylvania School of Dental Medicine in 2000. He subsequently completed his oral medicine fellowship and oral biology training at Harvard School of Dental Medicine. He is board certified in oral medicine and practices at Brigham and Women's Hospital and Dana-Farber Cancer Institute with special interest in oral mucosal diseases, salivary gland diseases, and oral complications in cancer patients. He is an assistant professor of oral medicine in the Department of Oral Medicine, Infection and Immunity at Harvard School of Dental Medicine, where he is the program director of postgraduate oral medicine.

Acknowledgments

We would like to thank Eric Stoopler, Mark Lerman, Ross Kerr, Andres Pinto, Juan Yepes, Vidya Sankar, Raj Lalla, Kevin Emerick, Francisco Marty, Dena Fischer, and Elaine Crooks for their critical and constructive comments on the text. We are indebted to Mark Lerman, Andres Pinto, Sook-Bin Woo, Stephen Sonis, Ross Kerr, Mark Schubert, Ellen Eisenberg, Michael Pharoah, and Scott De Rossi for their generous contributions of clinical images. We are particularly grateful to our administrative and clinical coworkers and professional colleagues for their continued dedication and drive towards excellence in patient care. We extend our gratitude to our mentors and colleagues who have provided invaluable insight, guidance, and inspiration, and to our students and residents for their continuous enthusiasm for knowledge and growth. Most importantly, we cannot forget our patients and their families, many of whom we will never forget, for putting their trust in our care. And last, but not least, we extend a very warm thanks to our loving families for their unconditional support of our professional and academic pursuits.

Jean Bruch, DMD, MD
Nathaniel Treister, DMD, DMSc

Contents

Chapter 1
Normal Anatomy

Summary Knowledge of normal anatomy and physiology of the oral cavity provides a basis for understanding and recognizing pathology. This chapter provides a review and overview of surface landmarks and underlying anatomy of the oral cavity in the context of diagnosing conditions that are detailed throughout the remainder of the book. The oral mucosa, palate, tongue, floor of mouth, dentition, salivary glands, and cervical lymphatic drainage are specifically highlighted.

Keywords Vermillion • Vestibule • Oral cavity proper • Oropharynx • Fauces • Palatoglossal arch • Palatopharyngeal arch • Retromolar trigone • Pterygomandibular raphe • Buccinator muscle • Muscles of mastication • Stenson duct • Wharton duct • Waldeyer ring • Lingual papillae • Tonsils • Tongue • Palate • Mucosa • Floor of mouth • Mucogingival junction • Parotid papilla • Palatal rugae • Periosteum • Gingival margin • Interdental papilla • Cementoenamel junction • Cementum • Enamel • Pulp • Foramen cecum • Incisive papilla • Apical foramen • Periodondal ligament • Trigeminal nerve • Temporomandibular joint • Parotid gland • Submandibular gland • Sublingual gland • Minor salivary glands • Lingual nerve • Inferior alveolar nerve • Cervical lymph nodes

1.1 Introduction

The oral cavity sits at the opening of the digestive tract and is bounded by the lips anteriorly (Fig. 1.1). The vermillion zone serves as the transition area between the moist oral mucosa and the skin of the face. The oral structures are adapted to serve a variety of functions, including maintenance of a protective barrier, initiation of digestion, special taste sensation, speech and swallowing, immunologic defense, and provision of salivary lubricants and buffers.

1.2 Surface Landmarks

The oral cavity can be subdivided broadly into three areas consisting of the vestibule, oral cavity proper, and oropharynx (Fig. 1.2). The *vestibule* is the space that is present between the lips or cheeks laterally and the dentition medially. The *oral cavity proper* lies inside the dental arches and is bounded posteriorly by the anterior pillar of the fauces, or *palatoglossal arch*. The *oropharynx* lies posterior to the palatoglossal arch, and includes the posterior one-third of the tongue, palatine tonsils, soft palate, and visible posterior wall (Fig. 1.3). The palatine tonsils sit in an alcove between the anterior (palatoglossal) and posterior (*palatopharyngeal*) arches, or *pillars*, and frequently exhibit surface pits or depressions called *crypts* (Fig. 1.4).

The *retromolar trigone* is a roughly triangular area behind the last molars representing the posterior aspect of the vestibule (Fig. 1.5). Adjacent to this is the *pterygomandibular raphe*, which indicates the junction between the buccinator and superior constrictor muscles, and is used as a landmark for administration of intraoral local anesthesia. The *parotid papilla*, which houses the opening of

J.M. Bruch and N.S. Treister, *Clinical Oral Medicine and Pathology,*
DOI 10.1007/978-1-60327-520-0_1, © Humana Press, a part of Springer Science+Business Media, LLC 2010

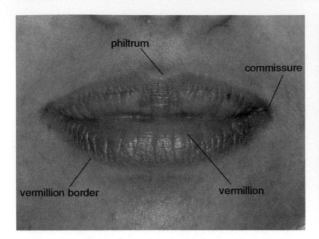

Fig. 1.1 Anatomy of the lips. Note small melanotic macule on the vermillion of the left upper lip near the border as well as physiologic pigmentation of upper lip

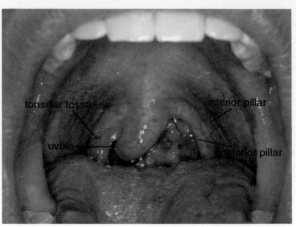

Fig. 1.3 Posterior oral cavity/oropharynx. The anterior pillar (*palatoglossal arch*) marks the posterior boundary of the oral cavity proper. The palatine tonsils, which are located in the tonsillar fossae, are not visible in this photo. *Asterisk* marks posterior oropharyngeal wall

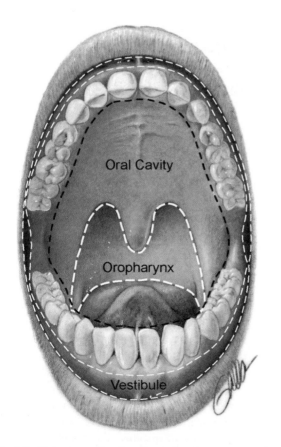

Fig. 1.2 Major areas of oral cavity: oral cavity proper, oropharynx, and vestibule. The vestibule is referred to as "buccal" posteriorly and "labial" anteriorly where it contacts the cheek and lip, respectively

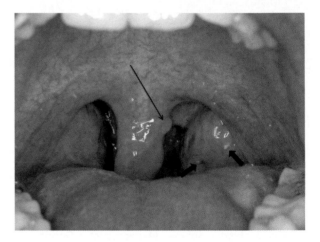

Fig. 1.4 Oropharynx showing large palatine tonsils with prominent crypts. Note debris visible within crypts on the left (*short arrows*) as well as a papilloma at the left base of uvula (*long arrow*)

Stenson duct of the parotid gland, is located in the buccal vestibule opposite the maxillary second molar (Fig. 1.6).

Folds of mucosa in the midline maxillary and mandibular labial vestibules can be seen anchoring the lips to the alveolar mucosa or gingiva, and are known as the *labial frenula* (Figs. 1.7 and 1.8). These can be quite prominent in some cases and even affect tooth eruption.

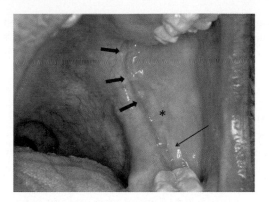

Fig. 1.5 Posterior oral cavity showing left retromolar trigone (*long arrow*) and pterygomandibular raphe (*short arrows*). Local anesthetic for a mandibular nerve block is injected lateral to the raphe, piercing the buccinator muscle (*asterisk*)

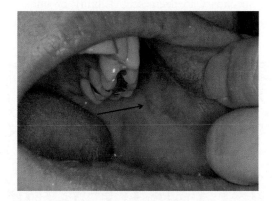

Fig. 1.6 Left maxillary buccal vestibule. Note parotid papilla with drop of saliva at opening of Stenson duct (*arrow*). Amalgam restorations are present in the maxillary posterior teeth

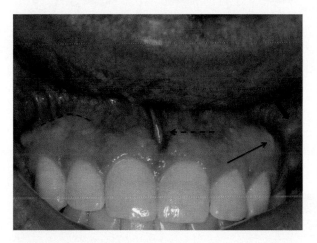

Fig. 1.7 Maxillary labial vestibule showing frenulum (*broken arrow*). Note bulge over root of canine tooth (canine eminence; *long solid arrow*) and adjacent depression (canine fossa; *short solid arrow*). A portion of the mucogingival junction is marked with a broken line on the right. Sebaceous glands are visible on the inner aspect of the upper lip

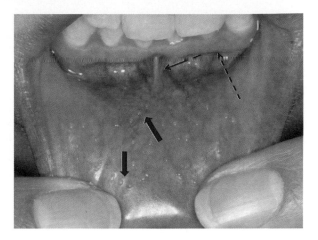

Fig. 1.8 Mandibular labial vestibule. Note frenulum (*long solid arrow*) and secretions from minor salivary glands in the lower lip (*short solid arrows*). The mucogingival junction represents the transition from thin nonkeratinized alveolar mucosa to the thicker keratinized attached gingiva and is quite prominent in this photo (*broken arrow*)

1.3 Oral Mucosa

The lining of the oral cavity serves a variety of functions, including protection, sensation, and secretion, and is histologically adapted to the unique environment inside the mouth. Oral mucosa lacks the appendages seen in skin, although sebaceous glands can be found in the upper lip and buccal mucosa in approximately 75% of adults (see Chap. 2). Submucosal minor salivary glands are found throughout the oral cavity, with highest concentrations in the palate and lower lip. Aggregates of lymphoid tissue can also be found in the oral cavity, however, the largest collection of lymphoid tissue is seen posteriorly and known as *Waldeyer ring*. This consists of the palatine, lingual, and adenoid (pharyngeal) tonsils, and virtually encircles the entrance to the oropharynx. Small nodules of accessory tonsil tissue are often seen on the posterior wall of the oropharynx and may become enlarged with inflammation or infection and mistaken for a suspicious mass. Normal pits and depressions in tonsil tissue (*tonsillar crypts*) may become plugged with keratin or other debris and form cysts which appear yellow to white in color (Figs. 1.4 and 1.9).

The majority of the oral cavity is lined by soft, moist, pliable, nonkeratinized mucosa which is loosely attached to underlying tissues and exhibits some mobility. This

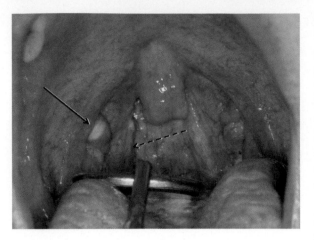

Fig. 1.9 Lobulated tonsils with cyst evident in the superior right tonsillar pole (*long solid arrow*). Note blunted and slightly bifid tip of uvula. Posterior pillar is marked with a *broken arrow*

consists of a stratified squamous epithelium which continually renews itself by division of progenitor cells in the deeper basal layer (Fig. 1.10). New cells show progressive maturation as they migrate to the surface layers, which are subsequently shed. Areas of the mouth that receive a greater degree of masticatory stress, namely the hard palate, tongue dorsum, and gingiva, are lined with keratinized mucosa, giving more protection against friction and abrasion. This tissue is more firmly attached to the underlying periosteum, which prevents damage from shearing forces.

The *mucogingival junction*, where the mobile mucosa lining the vestibule and floor of mouth joins the tightly adherent *gingiva* of the dental alveolus, should be easily visible in the healthy state. The gingiva appears paler pink secondary to decreased visibility of underlying blood vessels through the relatively opaque keratin

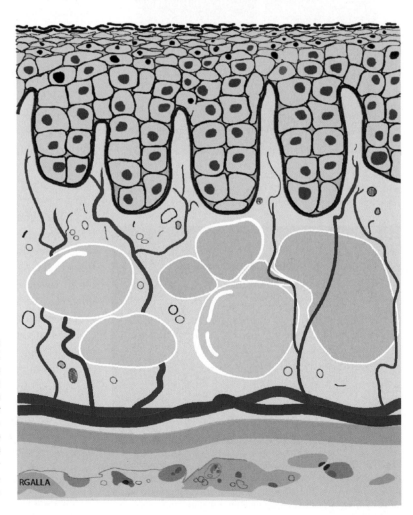

Fig. 1.10 Normal stratified squamous epithelium. The basal cells are cuboidal and abut the basement membrane. The shape becomes more flattened (squamoid) as the cells mature and move toward the surface. Irregularly shaped spinous, or prickle, cells are present in the intermediate layers. Surface keratin keratin is also present in this diagram. The connective tissue layer below the basement membrane contains blood vessels, lymphatics, fatty tissue, fibrous and elastic tissues, bone, and muscle

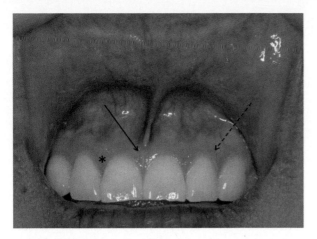

Fig. 1.11 Maxillary labial vestibule showing healthy appearing soft tissues with gingival stippling (*solid arrow*), rolled gingival margin (*broken arrow*), and sharp interdental papillae (*asterisk*). Note wear on incisal edges of maxillary central incisors

layer. The *gingival margin* should be well defined with slightly rolled margin and pointed interdental papillae. Healthy tissue will exhibit stippling, representing collagen fibers attaching the gingiva to the underlying periosteum (Figs. 1.7, 1.8, and 1.11).

1.4 Tongue

The tongue is divided into the *oral tongue* (anterior two-thirds) and *tongue base* (posterior third) by the *circumvallate papillae*, which form a v-shaped line anterior to the *foramen cecum* (Fig. 1.12). The foramen cecum is a shallow depression which exists as a developmental remnant of the thyroglossal duct. The oral tongue is typically subdivided into four areas: tip, lateral surfaces (sides), dorsum (top), and ventral (undersurface).

Embryologically, the mucosa lining the anterior portion of the tongue arises from the first branchial arch, and carries with it the trigeminal nerve. The mucosa of the tongue base arises from the third arch and is innervated by the glossopharyngeal nerve. The intrinsic muscles of the tongue are derived from the occipital somites, and are supplied by the hypoglossal nerve. Lingual tonsil tissue is frequently seen on the surface of the tongue posterior to the circumvallate papillae and lining the *vallecula*, which is a valley-like depression separating the tongue base from

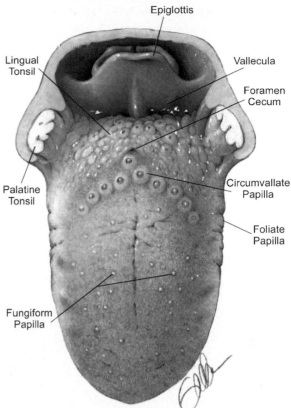

Fig. 1.12 Tongue dorsum showing major surface landmarks. (After Janfaza (2001) with permission; Lippincott Williams and Wilkins)

the epiglottis. Mucus glands are present posteriorly, and open into the crypts of the lingual tonsil.

The epithelium lining the tongue dorsum is specialized to withstand masticatory trauma as well as receive taste sensation. The dorsum has an irregular, bumpy, surface secondary to the presence of *papillae*. Although some taste receptors (*taste buds*) can be found in the soft palate and pharynx, the majority are located on the lingual papillae. Numerous small, hair-like, keratinized, *filiform papillae* cover the anterior surface of the tongue dorsum and do not contain taste receptors. These projections provide an abrasive surface that helps break down food against the hard palate during mastication. They are interspersed with fewer numbers of larger, smooth, and more rounded nonkeratinized *fungiform papillae,* with taste buds present on their superior surface. The fungiform papillae frequently appear deeper red in hue compared to the filiform papillae, as the color of the underlying vascular core is transmitted prominently through the epithelium (Fig. 1.13). *Foliate papillae* are ridge-like structures on the posterolateral aspect of the tongue containing taste buds on their lateral surfaces, and are often mistaken for abnormal tissue on oral exam. They vary greatly in size, and are virtually absent in some patients (Fig. 1.14). The *circumvallate papillae* are large round structures on the posterior tongue dorsum which also house taste buds. These are usually not appreciated on exam unless the tongue is protruded, and are also sometimes mistaken for pathology (Fig. 1.13).

1.5 Floor of Mouth

The lateral and ventral surfaces of the tongue, as well as the floor of mouth, are lined by thin, smooth, nonkeratinized mucosa that is fairly translucent (Fig. 1.15). Veins along the ventral surface of the tongue are easily visualized through the mucosa and can be quite prominent. A fringed fold of mucosa, called the *plica fimbriata*, sits lateral to the midline on each side and frequently contains tissue tags that can be mistaken for pathology. The sublingual salivary glands can be palpated laterally and frequently will be seen to bulge into the floor of mouth. The main sublingual duct joins the submandibular (*Wharton*) duct to empty into the oral cavity at the sublingual papilla near the base of the lingual frenulum. Additional tiny ducts open from the sublingual gland directly into the overlying mucosa.

1.6 Palate

The palate forms the roof of the oral cavity and is divided into the *hard palate* anteriorly and the *soft palate* posteriorly (Figs. 1.16 and 1.17). The mucoperiosteum of the hard palate is tightly bound and immobile, which explains why dental injections into this area are especially painful. The midline *incisive papilla* anteriorly indicates the opening of the incisive canal, which transmits the sensory

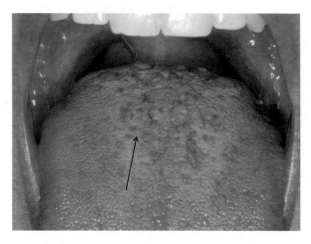

Fig. 1.13 Tongue dorsum showing contrast of fungiform papillae (*long arrow*) against background of lighter colored filiform papillae. Note row of circumvallate papillae (*short arrow*) posteriorly

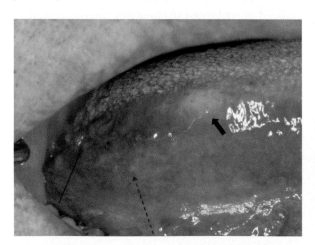

Fig. 1.14 Foliate papillae (*long solid arrow*). Also note prominent submucosal veins (*broken arrow*) and frictional hyperkeratosis (*short solid arrow*)

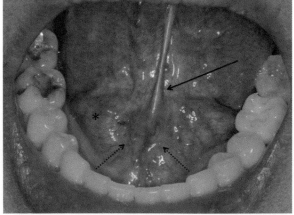

Fig. 1.15 Floor of mouth. Note frenulum (*solid arrow*), submandibular duct orifices (*broken arrows*), and visible prominence of sublingual gland under the mucosa (*asterisk*)

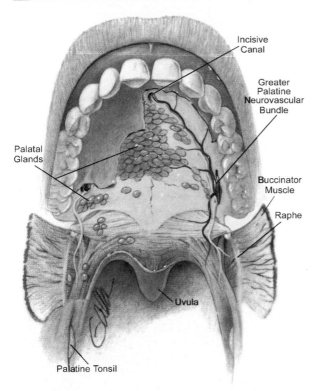

Fig. 1.16 Palate with cutaway view showing submucosal glands, musculature, and neurovascular bundles exiting the incisal and greater palatine foramina

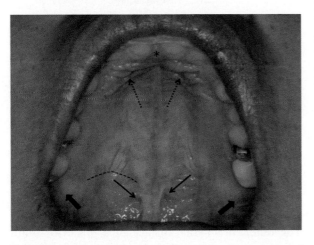

Fig. 1.17 Palate. Note junction of hard and soft palate (*dotted line*), maxillary tuberosities (*thick solid arrows*), palatine fovea (*thin solid arrows*), rugae (*broken arrows*), and incisive papilla (*asterisk*). The midline raphe is clearly evident

nasopalatine nerves to the anterior hard palate. A midline raphe can be visualized, representing embryologic fusion of the palatal shelves. Lateral

folds of mucosa, known as *palatal rugae*, are present anteriorly and assist in mastication. At the posterior aspect of the hard palate in the midline the palatine fovea can be seen as small pits, formed by coalescence of mucous gland ducts. The greater palatine neurovascular bundle exits its bony foramen under the mucosa opposite the maxillary second molar, innervating the posterior hard palate. The *maxillary tuberosity* can be palpated posterior and lateral to this behind the last molar, as the broad posterior extent of the maxilla.

1.7   Dentition

The tooth containing portion of the oral cavity is divided into maxillary and mandibular *dental arches* (Fig. 1.18). These are each further divided in half by the midline into *quadrants*. The teeth sit within the raised, *alveolar* (tooth bearing) *bone* of the dental arches. The adult, or secondary, dentition consists of 32 teeth, with 3 molars, 2 premolars ("bicuspids"), 1 canine ("eye tooth" or "cuspid"), and 2 incisors per quadrant. Molars and premolars are referred to as posterior teeth; canine and incisors are anterior. The pediatric, or primary, dentition contains a total of 20 teeth, with 2 molars, 1 canine, and 2 incisors per quadrant. The premolars erupt into the space occupied by the primary molars, and the permanent molars erupt posterior to this as the jaws and dental arches elongate with growth.

There are a variety of numbering systems used to identify each tooth. The most widely accepted method numbers the teeth from "1" to "32," beginning with the upper right third molar (tooth #1) and proceeding clockwise across the upper then lower arches, ending with the lower right third molar (tooth #32).

Each tooth consists anatomically of a *root* and *crown*, with the crown being the portion visible above the gingival margin (Fig. 1.19). The bulk of the tooth is made up of a calcified substance known as *dentin*, with an outer surface layer of harder *enamel* covering the crown and a softer material called *cementum* lining the root surface. The hollow inner core of the tooth, or *pulp chamber*, contains a soft jellylike material referred to as *pulp*, with nerve endings and blood vessels entering through the tip (*apex*) of the root via the *apical foramen*.

a

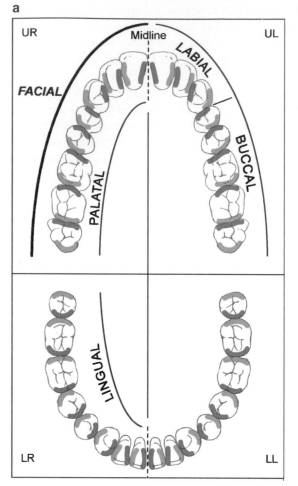

b

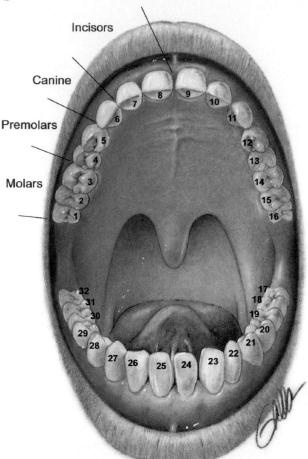

Fig. 1.18 Adult dentition. (**a**) Maxillary and mandibular dental arches. The four quadrants are referred to as upper right (*UR*), upper left (*UL*), lower left (*LL*), and lower right (*LR*). Mesial tooth surfaces are indicated in *blue*; distal in *pink*. The maxillary and mandibular dental midlines are marked with a *broken line*. The lingual, palatal, and facial

(which includes buccal and labial) surfaces are also indicated. (**b**) Commonly used numbering system for teeth, beginning with tooth #1 in the upper right quadrant and proceeding around the arches in a clockwise fashion. Each quadrant contains three molars, two premolars, one canine, and two incisors

The clinically visible junction of crown and root is called the *cementoenamel junction*, and is generally protected by the free upper edge of the gingival margin in the healthy state. Gingival recession may occur, with exposure of the softer root surface and concomitant increased risk of root surface caries, abrasion, or sensitivity. The tooth is anchored to the bony socket by collagen fibers (*periodontal ligament*), which can be weakened or destroyed by periodontal disease.

The crown of every tooth has five surfaces, and each one is specifically named. The biting surface

of a posterior tooth is referred to as the *occlusal* surface. The more tapered biting, or incising, surface of an anterior tooth is called the *incisal edge*. The outer, or lateral, surface of a posterior tooth adjacent to the cheek is referred to as *buccal*. The same surface of a more anterior tooth adjacent to the lip is *labial*. Alternatively, any buccal or labial surface may also be referred to as the *facial* surface. The inner, or medial, surface of a lower tooth abutting the tongue is *lingual,* and the same surface of an upper tooth facing the palate is *palatal*. The

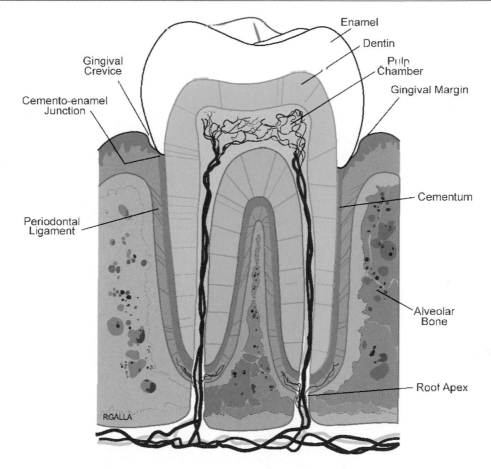

Fig. 1.19 Anatomy of a tooth. The cementoenamel junction represents the anatomic junction of the root and crown; this is also referred to as the "neck" or cervical area of the tooth. The apical foramen, which opens at the tip of each root, transmits the neurovascular bundle. (Reprinted with permission from Janfaza (2001); Lippincott Williams and Wilkins)

contacting surfaces of adjacent teeth are called *interproximal;* with the posteriorly oriented surface (i.e., away from midline) being *distal,* and the more anteriorly oriented surface (toward midline) being *mesial.*

1.8 Temporomandibular Joint

The temporomandibular joint (TMJ), where the football-shaped *condylar process* of the mandible articulates with the glenoid fossa of the temporal bone, is a synovial joint, and is located immediately anterior to the external auditory canal (Fig. 1.20). A roughly biconcave fibrocartilage disk (*meniscus*) is positioned within the joint space, dividing it into upper and lower cavities and allowing both hinge and gliding movements. The joint is enclosed by a fibrous capsule, and surrounding ligaments limit excessive joint movement. Dislocation of the jaw occurs when the mandibular condyle moves anterior to the *articular eminence.*

The initial 10–15 mm of mouth opening occurs by hinge-like *rotation* of the condyle against the articular disk in the inferior joint space without movement of the disk itself or movement in the upper joint space. With wider mouth opening, the superior surface of the disk then glides anteriorly downward along the articular eminence, carrying the condyle along with it. This second

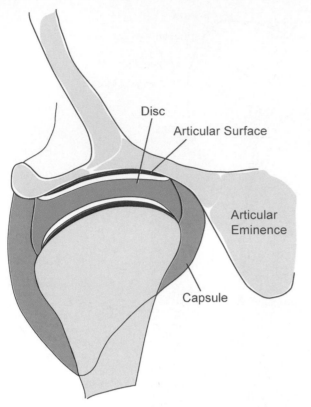

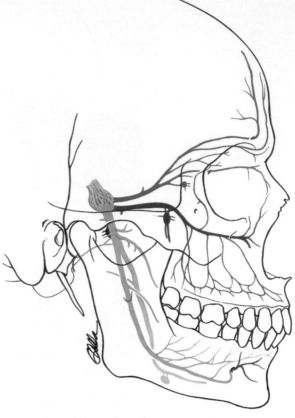

Fig. 1.20 Temporomandibular joint. Note how the mandibular condyle seats into the concave glenoid fossa of the temporal bone posterior to the articular eminence. The joint space is separated into superior and inferior spaces by the articular disk. In cases of internal derangement of the TMJ, the disk may be displaced anteriorly

Fig. 1.21 Trigeminal nerve showing the three divisions: V1 (*orange*), V2 (*green*), and V3 (*lavender*). (Reprinted with permission from Janfaza (2001); Lippincott Williams and Wilkins)

type of movement is referred to as *translation*. This sequence is then reversed with jaw closure.

Internal derangement of the joint can occur with destruction or detachment of the disk, in which case the disk may be displaced or dislocated (usually anteriorly, in front of the condyle). In patients with this problem, a "click" may be present upon mouth opening as the condyle moves forward during translation and spontaneously recaptures the disk. This is referred to as *reduction* of the disk, and a *reciprocal click* may be noted with closure as the condyle again moves posterior to the disk. In a situation where reduction does not occur, the disk can become jammed anterior to the condyle and limit the degree of mouth opening; in severe cases this can result in a *closed lock* with limitation of mouth opening.

1.9 Innervation

1.9.1 Jaws and Teeth

As first branchial arch derivatives, the maxilla and mandible are supplied by the trigeminal nerve (CN 5), which is predominantly sensory (Fig. 1.21; Table 1.1). The trigeminal (semilunar or Gasserian) ganglion is located in the floor of the middle cranial fossa and gives rise to three large nerve trunks. The *ophthalmic division* (V1) travels to the eye via the superior orbital fissure. The *maxillary division* (V2) passes through the foramen rotundum into the pterygopalatine fossa, where it receives sensory input from the maxillary alveolar bone, upper teeth, hard palate, and mucosa via

Table 1.1 Cranial nerves

Number	Name	Function(s)
I	Olfactory	Sense of smell
II	Optic	Vision
III	Oculomotor	Eye movement (except that mediated by lateral rectus and superior oblique muscles)
IV	Trochlear	Eye movement (mediated by superior oblique muscle)
V	Trigeminal	Oral/facial sensation; muscles of mastication
VI	Abducens	Eye movement (mediated by lateral rectus muscle)
VII	Facial	Facial sensation and taste (anterior tongue); muscles of facial expression and stapedius; and secretomotor innervation to salivary glands (except parotid)
VIII	Vestibulocochlear	Hearing and balance
IX	Glossopharyngeal	Sensation and movement of pharynx; taste to posterior tongue; and secretomotor innervation to parotid gland
X	Vagus	Main sensory and motor innervation to larynx and pharynx; taste sensation from epiglottis; and parasympathetic supply to thoracic and abdominal viscera
XI	Spinal accessory	Trapezius and sternocleidomastoid muscles
XII	Hypoglossal	Tongue movement

the *posterior* and *anterior superior alveolar nerves, nasopalatine nerve*, and *greater palatine nerve*. The *mandibular division* (V3) exits the skull base through the foramen ovale, passes through the infratemporal fossa, and provides sensory innervation to the lower jaw via the *inferior alveolar nerve* (IAN), *buccal nerve*, and *mental nerve*. The IAN is encased within the bone of the mandible below the roots of the posterior mandibular teeth and is subject to injury during third molar (wisdom tooth) extraction.

Taste buds are present in highest concentration at the base of the circumvallate papillae, and to a lesser extent around the fungiform papillae. There may also be scattered taste receptors on the foliate papillae and throughout the mucosa of the soft palate and epiglottis. Special sensory taste fibers travel through the chorda tympani branch of the facial nerve to join the lingual nerve, providing taste sensation to the anterior two-thirds of the tongue. Special taste fibers to the posterior tongue travel with the glossopharyngeal nerve.

1.9.2 Tongue

The *lingual nerve* branches off from the mandibular division of the trigeminal nerve near the inner ramus of the mandible and supplies general sensation (pain, touch, and temperature) to the mucosa of the tongue anterior to the circumvallate papillae, floor of mouth, and mandibular anterior lingual gingiva. This nerve can be injured during third molar extraction or procedures involving the floor of mouth such as removal of a submandibular duct stone. The tongue base receives sensory input via the glossopharyngeal nerve (CN 9), except for a small area posteriorly supplied by CN10. Motor innervation to the intrinsic tongue muscles is supplied by the hypoglossal nerve.

1.9.3 Muscles of Mastication and Facial Muscles

The primary muscles of mastication include the *masseter, temporalis, lateral (external) pterygoid*, and *medial (internal) pterygoid* (Fig. 1.22). The lateral pterygoid functions in mouth opening and mandibular protrusion, whereas the other muscles act mainly to close the mouth. These muscles are innervated by motor branches of the trigeminal nerve, which arise from the mandibular division (V3). It is important to remember that other muscles, such as the strap muscles of the neck, affect mandibular position and function. Effective mastication also requires adequate function of muscles controlling the tongue, lips, and cheeks.

a

b

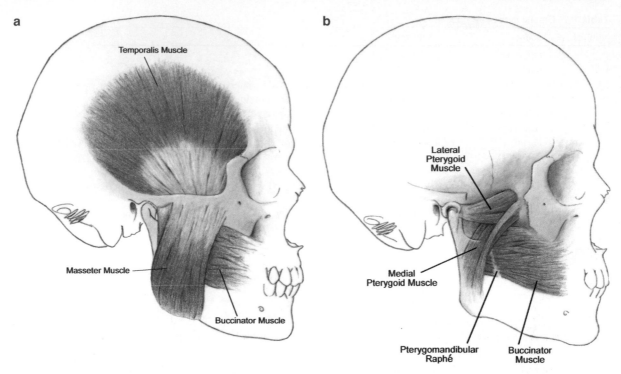

Temporalis Muscle

Lateral
Pterygoid
Muscle

Masseter Muscle

Buccinator Muscle

Medial
Pterygoid Muscle

Pterygomandibular
Raphé

Buccinator
Muscle

Fig. 1.22 Muscles of mastication. (**a**) The masseter originates from the maxillary zygomatic process/arch and inserts onto the lower aspect of the lateral mandibular ramus and angle. The temporalis arises from the temporal fossa of the lateral skull and inserts onto the coronoid process and ascending ramus of the mandible. Note buccinator muscle extending forward from underneath the masseter. (**b**) The lateral pterygoid arises from

the pterygoid plate of the sphenoid bone and inserts onto the TMJ capsule and mandibular condyle. The medial pterygoid originates more medially on the pterygoid plate and inserts onto the medial surface of the mandibular ramus. In this diagram, the mandibular ramus is rendered partially transparent to visualize the muscle insertion. Note origin of the buccinator muscle from the posterior mandible/maxilla and pterygomandibular raphe

The muscles of facial expression, or mimetic muscles, insert into the dermis of the skin and control movement around the scalp, orbit, ear, mouth, nose, and neck. They are all innervated by the facial nerve (CN 7). The *orbicularis oris muscle* forms the major sphincter of the lips, allowing complex movement in this area. The *buccinator muscle* makes up the bulk of the cheek and joins the superior pharyngeal constrictor muscle in the posterior oral cavity at the pterygomandibular raphe. Facial nerve paralysis, such as Bell's palsy, may result in flaccidity of the buccinator muscle, with decreased ability to control food in the vestibule or problems with cheek biting.

1.10 Salivary Glands

There are three sets of paired major salivary glands: sublingual, submandibular, and parotid (Figs. 1.23 and 1.24). The *sublingual gland* is the smallest, and

rests on the mylohyoid muscle in the anterolateral floor of mouth immediately under the mucosa. The secretions of this gland are primarily mucinous, and are therefore more viscous than saliva produced by the parotid and submandibular glands. The *submandibular gland* is larger and occupies the submandibular triangle with extension of the gland over the posterior border of the mylohyoid muscle into the floor of mouth. The secretions from this gland are mixed seromucinous, with viscosity intermediate between those of the sublingual and parotid glands.

The *parotid gland* is the largest of the three major salivary glands and is located in front of the ear (preauricular region), with extension to the posterior belly of the diagastric muscle inferiorly and the masseter muscle anteriorly (Fig. 1.24). The "tail" of the gland extends posteriorly under the earlobe to the sternocleidomastoid muscle (SCM). The gland is divided into superficial and deep lobes by the plane of the facial nerve (CN 7), with extension of the deep

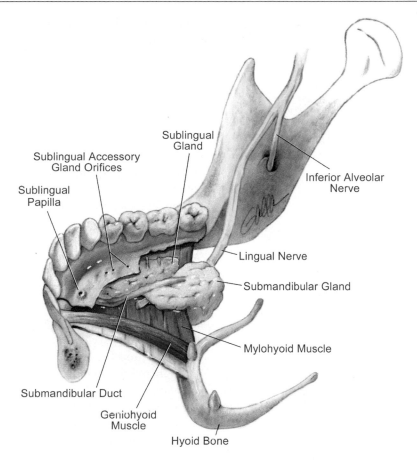

Sublingual Accessory Gland Orifices

Sublingual Papilla

Sublingual Gland

Inferior Alveolar Nerve

Lingual Nerve

Submandibular Gland

Mylohyoid Muscle

Submandibular Duct

Geniohyoid Muscle

Hyoid Bone

Fig. 1.23 Sublingual and submandibular salivary glands. The inferior alveolar nerve branches from the main trunk of V3 to enter the mandible on the medial surface of the ramus and travels forward within the bone to innervate the mandibular teeth; the small bump of bone illustrated adjacent to the foramen is called the *lingula*. The lingual nerve crosses from lateral to medial in the floor of mouth and passes underneath the submandibular duct prior to entering the tongue

lobe to the parapharyngeal space medially. Tumors of the deep lobe may result in visible bulging within the oral cavity in the region of the tonsil, and may present as the first sign of pathology. Lymph nodes are present within the parenchyma of the parotid gland, mainly in the superficial lobe, due to incorporation of lymphoid tissue into the gland during fetal development. These may present clinically as masses secondary to reactive or neoplastic processes. The parotid gland produces serous saliva, which is thin and watery compared to secretions from the other salivary glands.

There are hundreds of submucosal *minor salivary glands* present throughout the oral cavity (except for the gingiva and anterior hard palate), with a high density notable on the soft palate and posterolateral hard palate. Secretions from these glands are purely mucinous and represent a very small proportion of total salivary flow.

Innervation to the salivary glands is supplied by the autonomic nervous system, with both sympathetic and parasympathetic components. The parasympathetic system regulates fluid and electrolyte secretion, while the sympathetic system governs protein synthesis and secretion. The parotid gland receives parasympathetic secretomotor fibers from the glossopharyngeal nerve (CN 9), which synapse in the otic ganglion and then travel with the auriculotemporal branch of V3. Parasympathetic

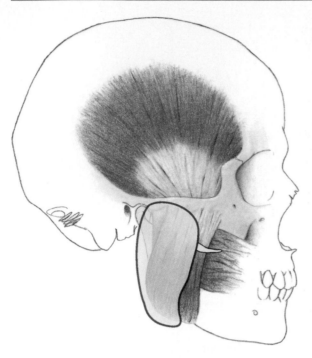

Fig. 1.24 Parotid gland schematically outlined overlying masseter muscle. The tail extends inferiorly below the angle of the mandible. The duct travels over the anterior edge of the masseter muscle then pierces the buccinator muscle to enter the oral cavity

fibers to the submandibular and sublingual glands travel with the facial nerve (CN 7) and chorda tympani to synapse in the submandibular ganglion prior to joining the lingual nerve. Sympathetic innervation to all of these glands is supplied from the superior cervical ganglion via the external carotid artery.

1.11   Lymphatics

Knowledge of lymphatic drainage pathways from the oral cavity and neck is important with respect to spread of infection and cancer (Fig. 1.25). The lymphatic system provides a mechanism to redirect tissue fluid back into the circulation, passing through a series of

lymph node "filters' along the way that function in immune surveillance.

Superficial cervical lymph nodes lie along the external and anterior jugular veins, superficial to the SCM muscle, receiving drainage from the skin of the scalp, face, neck, and ear. *Submental nodes* drain the chin, inner aspect of the lower lip, lower incisor teeth and gingiva, and tip of tongue. The submental nodes drain into *submandibular nodes*, which also receive drainage from the skin of the anterior face, anterior nasal cavity, anterior two-thirds of the tongue, and majority of dentition, gingiva, and hard palate.

The *deep cervical chain* of lymph nodes lies along the carotid sheath around the internal jugular vein extending from the base of skull into the root of the neck. These nodes are extremely important, as they ultimately receive all lymphatic drainage from the head and neck region. The *jugulodigastric node* drains the oropharynx, including tongue base, soft palate, and tonsils, and can be palpated just behind the angle of the mandible.

Drainage from tissues is generally to *ipsilateral* (same side) nodes, however, can cross over to the *contralateral* (opposite) side, particularly with midline structures. This is of particular concern in the case of the tongue, which has a very rich lymphatic supply. Progression of disease, such as inflammation, infection, or cancer, through the chain of cervical lymph nodes often occurs in predictable sequence. However, this is not always the case, as can be seen in patients with oral cancer which has spread to the neck and "skips over" certain groups of nodes.

Sources

Clemente C. Anatomy: A Regional Atlas of the Human Body. 5th ed. Lippincott, Williams and Wilkins; Baltimore, MD, 2007

Janfaza P. Surgical anatomy of the head and neck. Hagerstown, MD: Lippincott Williams and Wilkins, 2001

Jung HS, Akita K, Kim JY. Spacing patterns on tongue surface-gustatory papilla. Int J Dev Biol 2004;48:157–61

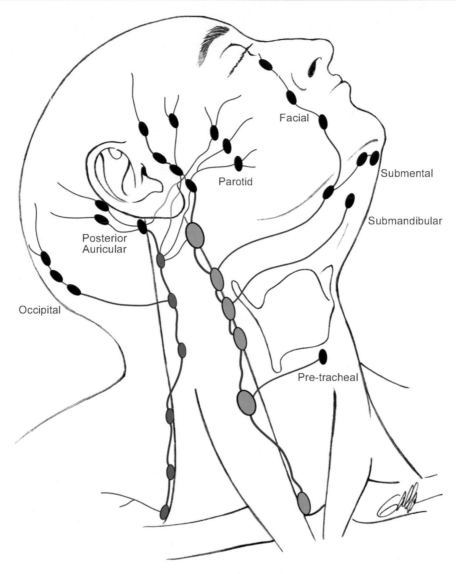

Fig. 1.25 Lymph nodes of the neck. The deep cervical chain is illustrated in *green*, which courses deep to the SCM at the level of the carotid sheath. The superficial cervical chain, which lies above the SCM, is illustrated in *blue*.

Kraus B, Jordan R, Abrams L. A Study of the Masticatory System; Dental Anatomy and Occlusion. Williams and Wilkins; Baltimore, MD, 1984

Netter F. Atlas of Human Anatomy. 4th ed. Saunders; Philadelphia, PA, 2006

Patil MS, Patil SB, Acharya AB. Palatine rugae and their significance in clinical dentistry: a review of the literature. J Am Dent Assoc 2008;139:1471–8

Pernkopf E. Atlas of Topographical and Applied Human Anatomy, 2nd ed. Vol. 1: Head and Neck. Munich: Urban and Schwarzenberg, 1980

Squier CA, Kremer MJ. Biology of oral mucosa and esophagus. J Natl Cancer Inst Monogr 2001;29:7–15

Thieme Atlas of Anatomy; Head and Neuroanatomy. Stuttgart: Georg Thieme Verlag, 2007

Chapter 2
Variants of Normal and Common Benign Conditions

Summary Fundamental to diagnosing oral pathologic conditions is the ability to recognize the spectrum of clinical findings that represents variation of normal within the population. The range of such variation is wide and findings can be very subtle or notably prominent. Some are purely developmental, while others have a clear inflammatory or traumatic etiology. This chapter describes the most commonly encountered variations of normal and benign conditions encountered in the oral cavity, with specific guidelines for diagnosis and management, when clinically indicated.

Keywords Melanocytes • Melanin • Physiologic pigmentation • Melanotic macule • Melanoma • Fordyce granule • Sebaceous gland • Gingival graft • Free gingival graft • Lingual tonsil • Tonsil • Fissured tongue • Geographic tongue • Benign migratory glossitis • Stomatitis erythema migrans • Erythema migrans • Median rhomboid glossitis • Fibroma • Irritation fibroma • Traumatic fibroma • Inflammatory papillary hyperplasia • Epulis fissuratum • Torus • Mandibular torus, • Maxillary torus • Exostosis • Ankyloglossia • Frenula

2.1 Introduction

Fundamental to diagnosing oral pathologic conditions is the ability to recognize the spectrum of clinical findings that represents variation of normal within the population. The range of such variation is wide and findings can be very subtle or notably prominent. Some are purely developmental, while others have a clear inflammatory or traumatic etiology. These conditions, in large part, do not require therapy unless specifically noted in the text.

2.2 Physiologic Pigmentation

Melanocytes are a normal component of the basal cell layer of the oral epithelium. They cause varying degrees of mucosal pigmentation, ranging from light brown to black, due to the production of melanin. *Physiologic pigmentation* is observed much more frequently in darker skinned individuals, however, even those with very fair complexions may demonstrate characteristic findings. Focal, freckle-like *melanotic macules* are very common (Fig. 2.1; see Chap. 6). The keratinized mucosa, in particular the gingiva, is most commonly affected (Fig. 2.2). Pigmentation is due to deposition of melanin into the connective tissue without an increase in the number or size of melanocytes, and lesions are therefore flat. This may become more pronounced in areas of chronic trauma or inflammation, such as along the occlusal bite line of the buccal mucosa (Fig. 2.3).

In most cases, the diagnosis can be made clinically but occasionally a biopsy is warranted to rule out melanoma; particularly if any changes are noted in size, shape, or degree of pigmentation, or if a flat lesion becomes raised. Intraoral melanoma, however, is exceedingly rare, representing less than 1% of all melanomas. Other causes of pigmentation, including both intrinsic and extrinsic etiologies, are discussed in Chap. 6.

> **Diagnostic tests**: None.
> **Biopsy**: No, with rare exception.
> **Treatment**: None.
> **Follow-up**: Annual.

J.M. Bruch and N.S. Treister, *Clinical Oral Medicine and Pathology*,
DOI 10.1007/978-1-60327-520-0_2, © Humana Press, a Part of Science + Business Media, LLC 2010

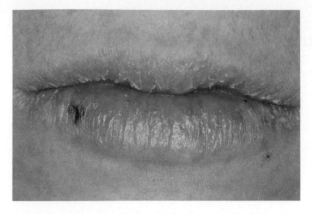

Fig. 2.1 Melanotic macule of the lower lip with dark brown pigmentation and sharply defined borders. The lips are slightly chapped.

2.3 Fordyce Granules

Sebaceous glands, which are a normal feature of facial skin, can often be identified within the buccal mucosa due to the proximity of skin to the oral mucosa in this area. These are less commonly noted on the lip or the labial mucosa (Figs. 2.4 and 2.5). Fordyce granules appear white to yellow in color, are generally present in clusters, may be slightly raised, and are asymptomatic. Sebaceous glands in the oral mucosa are nonfunctional. Occasionally patients become aware of

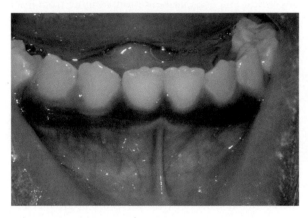

Fig. 2.2 Physiologic pigmentation in an African-American child. The interdental papillae are affected to a variable degree; the nonkeratinized mucosa is entirely unaffected.

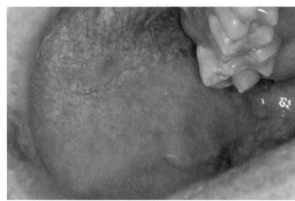

Fig. 2.4 Prominent Fordyce granules in the right buccal mucosa.

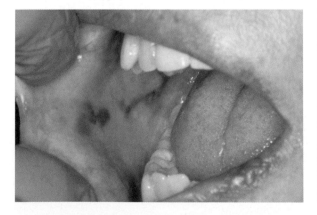

Fig. 2.3 Postinflammatory pigmentation of the right buccal mucosa secondary to chronic cheek biting.

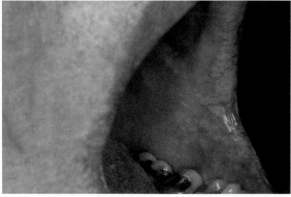

Fig. 2.5 Dense concentration of Fordyce granules in the left buccal mucosa.

their presence by detecting the raised surfaces with their tongue, or during self-examination with a mirror.

Diagnostic tests: None; clinical appearance is usually classic and sufficient for diagnosis.
Biopsy: No.
Treatment: None.
Follow-up: None.

2.4 Gingival Grafts

In cases of severe gingival recession, gingival grafting is performed as a periodontal surgical procedure to restore the attached soft tissue, reduce root-surface sensitivity, and prevent further tissue loss. The donor tissue, which is harvested from the patient's palate as an autograft, has a distinct appearance that is typically raised and more pale than the adjacent gingiva. Grafts are generally easily recognized, very sharply defined, and should not be mistaken for pathology (Fig. 2.6). If there is any doubt, the patient should be able to provide suitable history regarding whether such a procedure was performed.

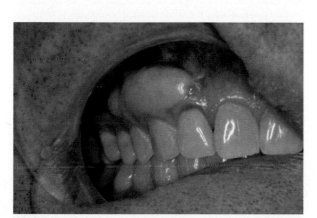

Fig. 2.6 Free gingival graft covering a prominent exostosis in an area of previous gingival recession. Note the thicker, more clearly defined keratinized mucosa compared to the adjacent nonkeratinized tissue.

Diagnostic tests: None.
Biopsy: No.
Treatment. None.
Follow-up: None.

2.5 Lingual Tonsil

Lymphoid tissue is often found along the posterior lateral tongue, forming part of *Waldeyer ring*. The clinical presentation ranges from imperceptible to strikingly prominent. Lingual tonsils appear as exophytic mucosal colored masses that may exhibit folds and crypts as seen in the palatine tonsils. As with any lymphoid tissue, these can become enlarged and tender secondary to inflammation. It is generally under these circumstances that patients or physicians become aware of their presence. Unilateral or asymmetrically enlarged tissue should be considered for biopsy to rule out other pathology such as lymphoma or squamous cell carcinoma.

Diagnostic tests: None.
Biopsy: No, unless unilateral or otherwise suspicious.
Treatment: None.
Follow-up: None.

2.6 Fissured Tongue

There is remarkable variation in the appearance of the tongue throughout the population. One common finding is the presence of fissures and grooves along the dorsal surface. These can range from shallow-appearing cracks to deep, penetrating fissures (Fig. 2.7). These features may be associated with geographic tongue (see below) and may rarely predispose to recurrent candidiasis (see Chap. 7). Most patients are universally asymptomatic; it is not uncommon for a patient to examine his or her tongue and become aware of fissuring following the onset of otherwise unrelated symptoms, such as burning mouth syndrome (see Chap. 10).

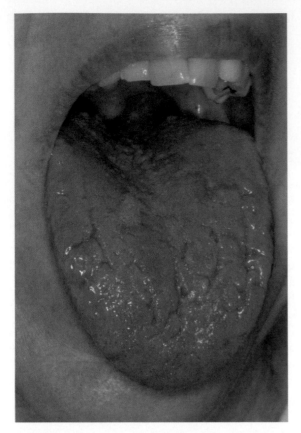

Fig. 2.7 Fissured tongue with extensive grooves and fissures over the entire dorsal surface.

Diagnostic tests: None.
Biopsy: No.
Treatment: None.
Follow-up: None.

2.7   Geographic Tongue

Also referred to as *benign migratory glossitis*, geographic tongue is a common inflammatory condition of the tongue. Other oral mucosal sites can be affected less frequently, in which case the condition is called *stomatitis erythema migrans* or *ectopic geographic tongue*. Geographic tongue is usually evident in early childhood and rarely causes symptoms. The lesions demonstrate a wide variety of clinical patterns, ranging from irregularly shaped erythematous macules with surrounding elevated white borders to patchy areas of depapillation and smooth glossy mucosa (Figs. 2.8–2.11). These fea-

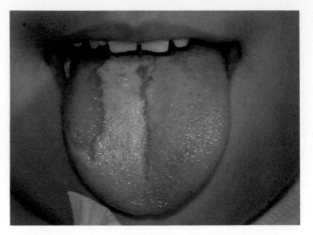

Fig. 2.8 Benign migratory glossitis in a child. There is a very well-defined area of depapillation on the right side of the tongue dorsum, while the rest of the surface is unaffected.

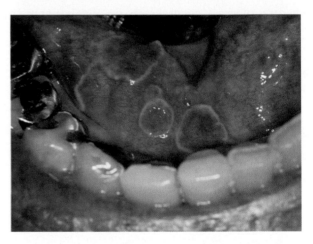

Fig. 2.9 Benign migratory glossitis of the ventral tongue and floor of mouth. As this region of the tongue does not normally contain papillae, only the white rimmed borders are noted.

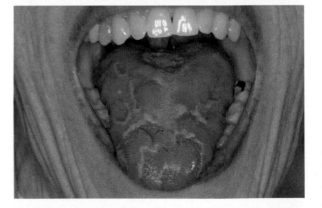

Fig. 2.10 Extensive benign migratory glossitis affecting the entire tongue dorsum with prominent areas of depapillation surrounded by white rimmed borders.

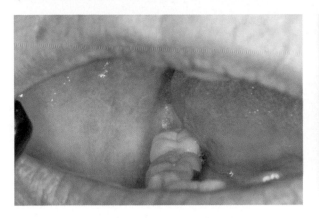

Fig. 2.11 Stomatitis erythema migrans showing subtle circular lesions with white borders of the right buccal mucosa and concurrent changes consistent with benign migratory glossitis.

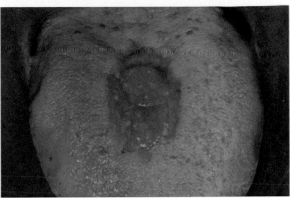

Fig. 2.12 Median rhomboid glossitis with a well-defined depapillated patch in the posterior midline of the tongue dorsum with normal surrounding tissue.

tures can give the tongue a map-like appearance, thus the descriptive term "geographic." In an affected individual, the presentation can change on a daily basis and therefore appear "migratory." Although the clinical presentation can be striking, there are few if any other conditions that mimic geographic tongue (these include oral lichen planus, erythematous candidiasis, and leukoplakia), and with a good history and examination lesions rarely warrant biopsy.

Albeit rare, patients may describe sensitivity of the tongue to otherwise normally tolerated food and beverages. This may or may not correlate with the extent of lesions noted clinically. Management with topical therapies may be effective in such cases. Importantly, other causes of tongue sensitivity must be considered, such as candidiasis or immune-mediated conditions, especially when there is recent or abrupt onset of symptoms.

> **Diagnostic tests**: None; diagnosis is based on clinical appearance.
>
> **Biopsy**: No, except very atypical presentations.
>
> **Treatment**: None in most cases. When symptomatic, rinses containing topical dexamethasone or diphenhydramine may be effective in reducing symptoms. Be sure to consider other causes of tongue discomfort, such as *burning mouth syndrome* (see Chap. 10).
>
> **Follow-up**: None.

2.8 Median Rhomboid Glossitis

This is a poorly understood condition that affects the tongue dorsum. It is characterized by a chronic, atrophic, erythematous, depapillated patch in the posterior midline of the tongue dorsum typically measuring between 0.25 and 2.0 cm in diameter (Fig. 2.12). While there is great variation in clinical presentation among patients, the size and quality of the lesion do not tend to change significantly over time in a given individual.

While many cases are never symptomatic, mild discomfort may develop specifically in the area of atrophic change. If so, symptoms tend to come and go and rarely persist for long. Because tissue biopsy often demonstrates superficial candidal colonization and an inflammatory infiltrate in the underlying connective tissue, there is some thought that median rhomboid glossitis is mediated by chronic candidal colonization. The tissue may be particularly susceptible to recurrent fungal infection due to the reduced thickness of the epithelium. Therefore, when a patient develops symptoms of tongue discomfort in the presence of median rhomboid glossitis, first-line treatment consists of topical or systemic antifungal therapy. If symptoms persist following an appropriate course of antifungal therapy, topical corticosteroid therapy should be instituted. If this is also ineffective and all other potential etiologies have been excluded, the discomfort should be managed as a neuropathic pain disorder (see Chap. 10).

Diagnostic tests: None routinely. A positive fungal culture or cytological smear may or may not represent a true infection (see Chap. 3). This may be clinically useful to determine baseline status prior to initiating antifungal therapy.

Biopsy: No, except for atypical presentations.

Treatment: None in most cases. When symptomatic, initial therapy should consist of a 1-week course of either clotrimazole troches or fluconazole. Be sure to consider other causes of tongue discomfort, such as *geographic tongue* or *burning mouth syndrome*. If there is no improvement following 1 week of antifungal therapy, treatment with high potency topical corticosteroid gels (fluocinonide 0.05% or clobetasol 0.05%), two to three times daily, should be initiated. If this is also ineffective, consider treating as a neuropathic condition (see Chap. 10).

Follow-up: None if asymptomatic, otherwise patients should be re-evaluated after 1 week of antifungal therapy.

2.9 Fibroma

Fibromas are probably the most commonly encountered oral soft tissue lesions. Frequently used terms include *irritation fibroma* and *traumatic fibroma*, indicating the underlying reactive etiology. These are initiated by trauma, typically a bite injury (that the patient may not recall) or secondary to friction from the sharp edge of a tooth or dental restoration. Fibromas present clinically as round or ovoid, firm, exophytic, smooth-surfaced masses that are the same color as, or slightly lighter than, the surrounding mucosa (Fig. 2.13). Lesions range in size from several millimeters to 1.0 cm in diameter (Fig. 2.14). Larger lesions are exceedingly rare and biopsy should be considered in such cases to rule out a neoplasm. As these are often caused by bite trauma, the most commonly involved areas are along the bite plane of the buccal mucosa and lateral tongue, although the lower labial mucosa and tongue dorsum can also be affected. There are no specific risk factors other than a history of minor trauma.

Fibromas are generally asymptomatic and do not require treatment unless they are particularly bothersome to the patient. Depending on the size and location, lesions may simply be an annoyance, or they may become quite uncomfortable due to repetitive trauma. Lesions may progressively enlarge with recurrent injury, thereby compounding the clinical situation. In such cases the surface mucosa often becomes ulcerated, characterized by a yellowish white pseudomembrane (Fig. 2.15).

Treatment is surgical excision, after which lesions rarely recur. Histopathological examination demonstrates a dense collection of fibrous tissue with normal surface epithelium. Fibromas have no malignant potential; however, they should be excised and submitted for histopathological analysis if the clinical diagnosis is uncertain.

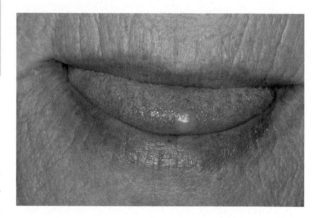

Fig. 2.13 Fibroma of the anterior tongue tip secondary to bite trauma. The lesion is well-defined and has a smooth, raised surface in comparison to the adjacent tissue; it is firm and nontender.

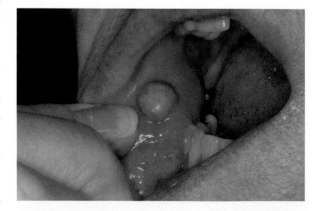

Fig. 2.14 Large fibroma of the right buccal mucosa. The surface mucosa is thicker in appearance than the surrounding tissue.

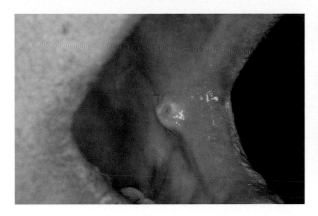

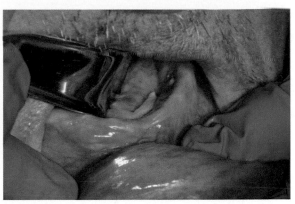

Fig. 2.15 Fibroma of the left buccal mucosa with focal ulceration secondary to repetitive bite injury.

Fig. 2.16 Fibrous hyperplasia of the mandibular mucosa secondary to a poorly fitting denture. Note the folds of dense fibrous tissue in the anterior floor of mouth (*epulis fissuratum*).

> **Diagnostic tests**: None.
> **Biopsy**: Only if the appearance is suspicious.
> **Treatment**: None if asymptomatic; otherwise complete surgical excision.
> **Follow-up**: None.

2.10 Inflammatory Papillary Hyperplasia

This is a benign reactive condition that develops on denture-bearing mucosa. This includes the maxillary and mandibular alveolar mucosa, the hard palate, and the vestibular mucosa. It only affects denture wearers and not patients who wear other removable oral appliances. Inflammatory papillary hyperplasia can affect a very limited area of mucosa or be quite extensive, in some cases involving the entire hard palate. A focal lesion with a distinct wrinkled or folded appearance is often termed *epulis fissuratum*, and is most commonly encountered in the anterior buccal vestibule at the edge of a denture flange (Fig. 2.16). Lesions are characterized by pebbly, papillary changes that are variably associated with tissue hyperplasia, and verrucous-like changes that can be quite notable (Fig. 2.17). This condition is rarely symptomatic, however, patients are typically aware of its presence. Depending on the location and extent of tissue hyperplasia, lesions may be susceptible to secondary trauma or interfere with prosthesis fit and function (Fig. 2.18).

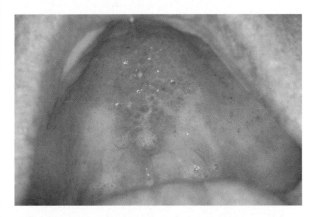

Fig. 2.17 Inflammatory papillary hyperplasia in a patient with a full upper denture. A punch biopsy was obtained to rule out malignancy. As the lesion was asymptomatic and the denture was otherwise comfortable, no further treatment was necessary.

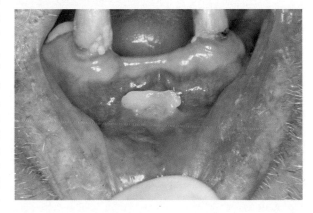

Fig. 2.18 Ulcerated epulis fissuratum due to a poorly fitting removable partial denture.

The etiology of inflammatory papillary hyperplasia is poorly understood. It is thought that chronic irritation due to a loose or poorly fitting denture, or inadequate denture hygiene (with candida colonizing the denture material), contributes to localized inflammatory-mediated reactive changes in the mucosa. As lesions may mimic other pathologic conditions, including *proliferative verrucous leukoplakia* and *squamous cell carcinoma* (see Chap. 9), biopsy may be necessary to rule out dysplasia or malignancy. Histopathological findings include benign papillary acanthosis (increased epithelial thickness) that is commonly associated with a chronic inflammatory infiltrate in the underlying connective tissue.

The first step in treatment is careful evaluation of the prosthesis. The extension of the denture borders into the vestibule as well as overall stability should be examined closely by an appropriate specialist. Recommendation should be made to soak the prosthesis overnight in an over the counter denture disinfectant solution or prescription chlorhexidine gluconate 0.12%. Another simple and inexpensive option for nonmetal containing prostheses is use of a 1:10 dilution of sodium hypochlorite, or common household bleach. Even in the absence of obvious oral fungal infection, a 1–2-week course of fluconazole 100 mg once daily, in addition to daily denture hygiene, is reasonable empiric therapy. During this time, the prosthesis should be left out of the mouth as much as possible to avoid exacerbation of the lesion. Surgical excision is indicated for lesions that fail to respond to conservative therapy and are bothersome or interfere with function (Fig. 2.19).

Diagnostic tests: None.

Biopsy: Yes, to rule out malignancy if the clinical appearance is suspicious.

Treatment: Prosthesis should be evaluated for fit, stability, and hygiene and adjusted or otherwise managed appropriately. Hyperplastic tissue can be surgically excised or laser ablated if bothersome or otherwise symptomatic.

Follow-up: None. Patients should be instructed to maintain good denture hygiene and return to their dentist for regular follow-up.

2.11 Tori and Exostoses

These are benign, developmental bony growths that are commonly observed in the oral cavity. Tori are more common and are specific to the midline hard palate and anterolateral lingual mandible. Similar lesions involving the buccal aspect of the maxilla or mandible are called exostoses. These areas are covered by keratinized or nonkeratinized mucosa, depending on the anatomic location, and can be mistaken for mucosal growths. Changes are not typically evident until the second decade, and while highly variable, growth is generally very slow throughout life. Even when lesions become quite extensive, patients may be unaware of their presence due to the gradual incremental growth pattern over decades.

Maxillary tori occur in the midline of the hard palate and range from barely discernable dome-shaped smooth swellings to large multilobulated masses (Figs. 2.20–2.22). Mandibular tori develop most commonly along

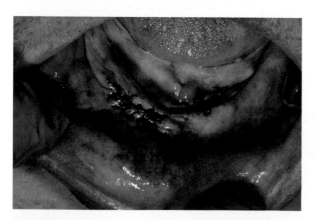

Fig. 2.19 Areas of fibrous tissue shown in Fig. 2.16 were excised and submitted for histopathology in preparation for fabricating a new set of complete dentures.

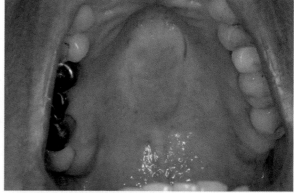

Fig. 2.20 Maxillary torus with smooth surface and well-defined borders in the midline of the hard palate.

the lingual aspect of the mandible inferior to the premolars bilaterally. Mandibular tori also exhibit a wide range of presentations; however, lesions usually demonstrate two to three well-defined smooth lobules (Fig. 2.23). Exostoses appear clinically identical to mandibular tori on the buccal surface of the mandible or maxilla (Fig. 2.6). These can grow to be quite large yet rarely have any discernable effect on the external facial appearance. On intraoral periapical dental radiographs, the involved areas appear as dense radiopacities within the maxilla and mandible (Fig. 2.24).

Tori and exostoses generally do not require any treatment. The covering mucosa may occasionally become irritated or ulcerated secondary to trauma, which is managed symptomatically. If denture fabrication is required, tori can be surgically removed to maximize retention of the prosthesis and minimize the risk of pressure-induced trauma.

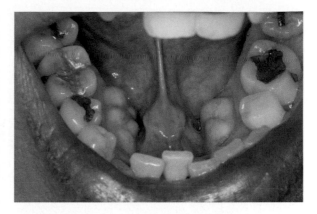

Fig. 2.23 Mandibular tori in the premolar region with multiple lobules.

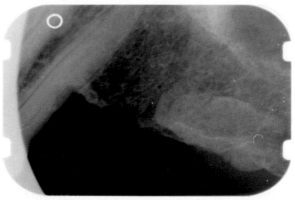

Fig. 2.24 Radiographic appearance of a maxillary torus as a well-defined radiopacity.

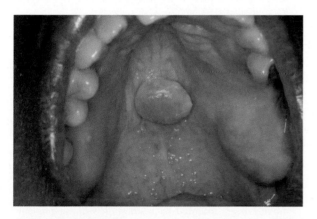

Fig. 2.21 Maxillary torus with a stalk-like attachment to the underlying palatal bone.

Diagnostic tests: None.
Biopsy: No.
Treatment: None.
Follow-up: None.

2.12 Ankyloglossia and Prominent Frenula

Abnormal prominence of *frenula* (tissue attachments of the anterior tongue and labial mucosa), can result in a variety of complications. In the case of the *lingual frenulum*, this can lead to problems with speech development or infant feeding, and is referred to *ankyloglossia* or "tongue tie." Localized periodontal recession on the lingual aspect of the central incisors can also occur. A prominent *labial mandibular frenulum* can

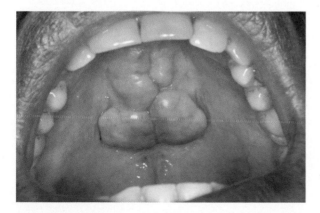

Fig. 2.22 Multilobulated maxillary torus showing slight asymmetry.

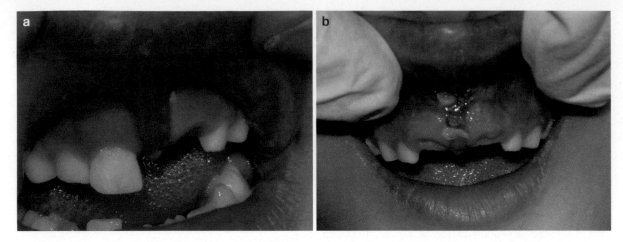

Fig. 2.25 Thick maxillary frenulum in a 5-year-old before (**a**) and after (**b**) surgical repositioning.

similarly affect the facial aspect of the same teeth. High insertion of the *maxillary frenulum* onto the gingiva may lead to formation of a gap, or *diastema*, between the central incisors (Fig. 2.25). These conditions are typically identified in young children by their dentist or pediatrician. If indicated, treatment is simple surgical repositioning or excision.

Diagnostic tests: None.
Biopsy: No.
Treatment: Referral to an oral surgeon that specializes in pediatrics for surgical evaluation.
Follow-up: None.

Sources

Antoniades DZ, Belazi M, Papanayiotou P. Concurrence of torus palatines with palatal and buccal exostoses: case report and review of the literature. Oral Surg Oral Med Oral Pathol Oral Radiol Endod 1998;85:552–7

Assimakopoulos D, Patrikakos C, Fotika C, et al. Benign migratory glossitis or geographic tongue: an enigmatic oral lesion. Am J Med 2002;15:751–5

Rogers RS, Bruce AJ. The tongue in clinical diagnosis. J Eur Acad Dermatol Venereol 2004;18:254–9

Canaan TJ, Meehan SC. Variations of structure and appearance of the oral mucosa. Dent Clin North Am 2005;49:1–14

Carter LC. Median rhomboid glossitis: review of a puzzling entity. Compendium 1990;11:446, 448–51

Cicek Y, Ertas U. The normal and pathological pigmentation of oral mucous membrane: a review. J Contemp Dent Pract 2003;15:76–86

Infante-Cossio P, Martinez-de-Fuentes R, et al. Inflammatory papillary hyperplasia of the palate: treatment with carbon dioxide laser, followed by restoration with an implant-supported prosthesis. Br J Oral Maxillofac Surg 2006; 45:658–60

Jainkittivong A, Langlais R. Geographic tongue: clinical characteristics of 188 cases. J Contemp Dent Pract 2005;6:123–35

Segal LM, Stephenson R, Dawes M, et al. Prevalence, diagnosis, and treatment of ankyloglossia; methodologic review. Can Fam Physician 2007; 53:1027–33

Chapter 3
Diagnostic Tests and Studies

Summary Diagnostic tests and studies often provide essential clinical data necessary to arrive at the correct diagnosis of various oral pathological conditions. In many cases, negative findings are just as revealing as positive findings. The most important considerations are when, why, and how to order certain studies, how to interpret the results, and what to do with the information obtained. This chapter emphasizes a rational approach to the utilization and interpretation of culture, imaging, and tissue-based diagnostic studies for the evaluation of patients with oral pathological conditions.

Keywords Saliva • Salivary glands • Culture • Herpes simplex virus • Varicella zoster virus • Direct fluorescence antibody test • Polymerase chain reaction • Cyto megalovirus • Radiographs • Computed tomography • Magnetic resonance imaging • Positron emission tomography • Ultrasonography • Scintigraphy • Sialography • Photography • Cytology • Fine needle aspiration biopsy • Biopsy • Direct immunofluorescence • Brush cytology • Toluidine blue

3.1 Introduction

When evaluating an oral medicine patient, obtaining a comprehensive yet targeted medical history and history of present illness is critical to generating a differential diagnosis. Key elements include: (a) medical conditions and comorbidities for which the patient is being treated; (b) medications and allergies; (c) whether this represents an initial or recurrent episode; (d) timing of oral symptoms and precipitating factors; (e) symptoms or lesions involving other areas of the body; (f) pain score if relevant; (g) whether the condition is improving, remaining stable, or getting worse; and (h) any treatments that have already been provided and their effectiveness. Throughout the following chapters, specific aspects of the history that are directly relevant to a particular condition or group of conditions are emphasized.

Diagnostic tests and studies often provide additional information necessary to arrive at the correct diagnosis. In many cases, negative findings are just as revealing as positive findings. The most important considerations are when, why, and how to order certain studies, how to interpret the results, and what to do with the information obtained. Throughout the following chapters, indicated studies are listed for each condition, and suggestions are made regarding interpretation of results within a specific clinical context.

3.2 Examination

The physical examination begins extraorally with visual inspection for evidence of extraoral lesions (e.g., erythema, rash, and pigmentation), asymmetry, and swelling. The head and neck should be carefully palpated for swelling, tenderness, and lymphadenopathy. The muscles of mastication (particularly the masseter and temporalis muscles) and the temporomandibular joint should be palpated for function and tenderness (see Chap. 10); any asymmetries, deviations to the left or right, or limitations in mouth opening should be noted. A cranial nerve examination should be performed to evaluate for neuromuscular and neurosensory deficits. If the patient reports any specific nonoral issues or findings these should also be investigated.

The entire oral cavity and oropharynx must be examined, regardless of the patient's chief complaint. A good light source is paramount. Any abnormalities of the soft tissue should be noted with respect to size,

J.M. Bruch and N.S. Treister, *Clinical Oral Medicine and Pathology,*
DOI 10.1007/978-1-60327-520-0_3, © Humana Press, a part of Springer Science+Business Media, LLC 2010

Table 3.1 Terms commonly used to describe oral lesions

Atrophy	Loss of tissue, typically due to thinning of cell layers; often associated with erythema
Bulla	A fluid-filled blister >0.5 cm in diameter
Ecchymosis	A macular area of submucosal hemorrhage (bruise) appearing as a well-defined area of erythema or purplish-blue pigmentation
Endophytic	A lesion that appears to be growing inward toward the underlying tissues
Erosion	Loss or thinning of superficial epithelial layers not extending through the full thickness of epithelium, typically secondary to inflammation
Erythema	Redness of the mucosa often due to a combination of inflammation, increased vascularity, and epithelial atrophy
Exophytic	A lesion that appears to be growing outward from the mucosa
Fixed	A lesion that is nonmobile and firmly attached to the underlying structures
Hematoma	A tumor-like collection of blood in the submucosa presenting as a well-defined raised lesion that is red, purple, or black
Indurated	Hard and firm upon palpation in tissue that would normally be soft
Leukoplakia	A white lesion that does not rub away and that cannot be defined by any obvious clinical entity; requires further evaluation to rule out potential malignancy
Macule	A well-defined flat lesion with color or texture changes
Mobile	A movable lesion that does not appear to be connected to underlying structures
Nodule	A solid mass visible or palpable within or underneath the mucosa
Papillary	A lesion with multiple finger-like projections
Papule	A well-defined elevated lesion <0.5 cm in diameter
Pedunculated	An exophytic lesion that is attached to the mucosa by a thinner stalk
Petechia	A small, punctate area of submucosal hemorrhage
Plaque	A well-defined elevated lesion >0.5 cm in diameter on skin or mucosal surface
Pustule	A small, well-defined accumulation of pus, usually located superficially
Sessile	An exophytic lesion that is firmly attached to the mucosa by a broad base
Ulcer	Loss of epithelium, typically presenting with a yellow or whitish-gray pseudomembrane
Vegetation	An exophytic lesion with multiple papillary or nodular areas of outgrowth
Verrucous	Papillary and deeply folded epithelial changes that can appear wart-like
Vesicle	A fluid-filled blister <0.5 cm in diameter

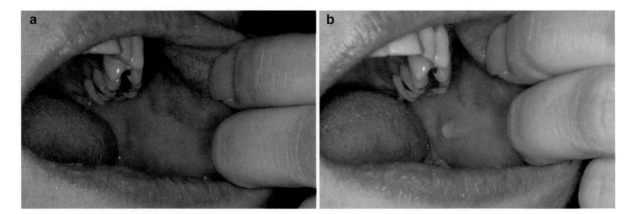

Fig. 3.1 Expression of serous saliva from the parotid gland duct orifice. (**a**) Saliva is seen as it begins to flow from Stenson's duct. (**b**) Expressed saliva flowing inferiorly toward the buccal vestibule

extent, thickness, texture, color, consistency, and tenderness (Table 3.1). The amount and consistency of saliva is observed, and the salivary gland duct orifices are evaluated for patency and flow (Fig. 3.1a and b). The dentition should be inspected for obvious *caries* (decay), fractured or missing restorations, excessive periodontal recession and bone loss (characterized by excessive root surface exposure), percussion sensitivity, mobility, and adjacent soft tissue swelling and/or purulent discharge (see Chap. 7). Removable prostheses should be evaluated for fit, comfort, and overall appearance and hygiene.

3.3 Culture Techniques

Microbial culturing is utilized to confirm (or rule out) the presence of an infection, to identify specific pathogens, and to determine antimicrobial susceptibilities. Understanding when to culture, which sampling technique to use, which culture techniques to request from the diagnostic laboratory, and how to properly submit the specimen are all critical to ensure that the culture yields useful diagnostic information.

3.3.1 Bacterial Cultures

There are remarkably few indications for obtaining bacterial cultures of the oral cavity, which is colonized in normal health with more than 300 species of commensal bacteria. Even when purulent material is drained from a dental abscess or suppurative bacterial parotitis is diagnosed, cultures are not typically submitted unless the condition does not respond to rational empiric antibiotic therapy in a timely manner. Both aerobic and anaerobic cultures should be collected by swabbing or aspirating the purulent material directly; culture and sensitivity testing should be requested. There are no generalized indications for surveillance mucosal swabbing.

3.3.2 Fungal Cultures

Similarly, fungal cultures of the oral cavity are not routinely obtained. *Candida albicans*, the most common fungal pathogen of the oral cavity, is a frequent component of normal oral flora. A positive culture is therefore not typically a useful or meaningful piece of information. Occasionally, a culture with antifungal susceptibilities may be indicated after a failed trial of empiric antifungal therapy in the presence of clinical signs of fungal infection.

3.3.3 Viral Cultures

In contrast to bacterial and fungal cultures, viral cultures are often a key diagnostic test when painful ulcers or lip crusting are present. Specific viral culture transport medium must be used and the specimen must be immediately transported to the laboratory, or kept on ice when on-site facilities are not available. Lesions are lightly swabbed with the sterile cotton tip which is then placed tip down into the medium and sealed (Fig. 3.2). Herpes simplex virus and Varicella zoster virus are both readily cultured from ulcerative lesions; although false negatives are common, particularly with resolving infections. Negative results require careful interpretation as the

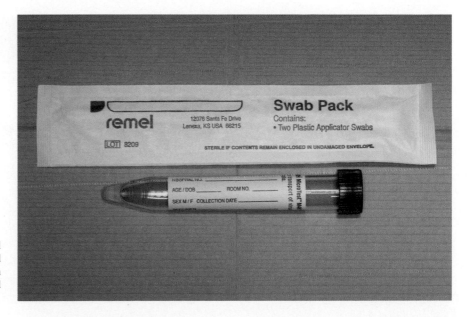

Fig. 3.2 Viral culture kit. Viral cultures can only be submitted in specific viral culture medium and must be kept on ice and processed in a timely manner

sample may have been inadequate or nonvital if there was a delay in transport/processing time, and reculturing should always be considered when there is continued clinical suspicion. DFA, or direct fluorescence antibody test, is a very rapid HSV test that requires a specific kit from the laboratory and is useful when an immediate (same day) diagnosis is required. Polymerase chain reaction (PCR) is an extremely sensitive assay that is increasingly being used; tests are available for most of the human herpes viruses. Herpesvirus PCR can be positive in the absence of clinical lesions secondary to asymptomatic viral shedding, thus caution should be used in interpreting results.

Cytomegalovirus (CMV), a rare cause of oral ulcers in immunocompromised patients, cannot be cultured from the surface exudate of ulcers as the virus resides deep in endothelial tissues. If CMV infection is suspected, an incisional biopsy of ulcerated tissue should be obtained and submitted for histopathology and viral isolation.

3.4   Blood Tests

Analysis of the blood and serum is often an important component of the diagnostic work-up of specific oral medicine conditions. Routinely ordered tests include complete blood count with white blood cell differential; iron, folic acid, and vitamin B12 levels; ANA, RF, SS-A, and SS-B levels; and antigen-specific antibody titers. Certain systemic medications used to treat oral

medicine conditions also require blood test monitoring for toxicity. Throughout the following chapters specific tests and their interpretation will be highlighted in the context of relevant medical conditions.

3.5   Radiographic Studies

Radiographic studies are utilized to image bony or mineralized lesions, determine the extent of soft tissue lesions, image the salivary glands, and evaluate lymph nodes. While there are no absolute guidelines, radiographic studies should be reserved for clinical situations where the information obtained will contribute to diagnosis, guide management, or allow evaluation of response to therapy.

3.5.1   Plain Films

Intraoral and extraoral plain film radiography provides a safe and inexpensive means of imaging the hard tissues of the maxilla and mandible. In most cases these images are acquired and interpreted at a clinical oral health facility rather than a hospital. Bitewing radiographs are useful for visualizing interproximal caries. Periapical radiographs are excellent for identifying periapical radiolucencies, which may be a sign of odontogenic infection (Fig. 3.3). Panoramic tomography

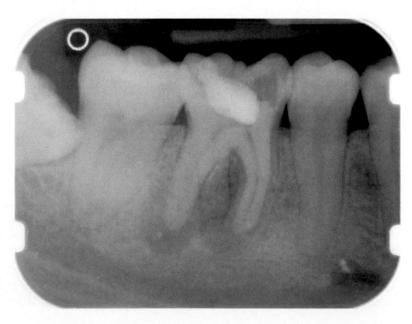

Fig. 3.3 Intraoral periapical radiograph. The position and resolution of this radiographic technique is optimal for evaluating the periapical region of teeth. In this case, dental caries have infected the pulp of the right mandibular first molar resulting in extensive periapical radiolucencies

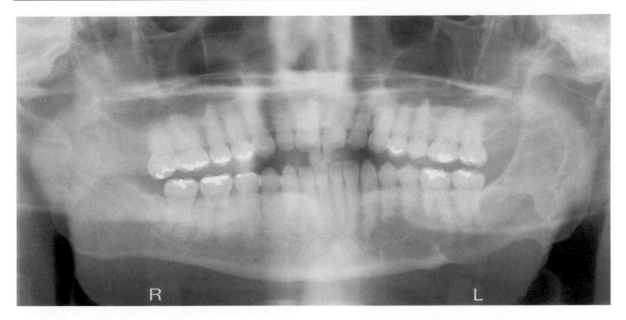

Fig. 3.4 Panoramic radiograph. This technique provides a complete image of the mandible and lower maxilla. In this case, a patient with multiple myeloma was evaluated for bisphosphonate-associated osteonecrosis of the *right* mandible and was found to have previously undiagnosed extensive myeloma involving the *left* ramus and body of the mandible

provides a complete image of the mandible and maxilla and is useful in evaluating expansile bony lesions. It can also be used as a method for imaging the dentition when the patient is not able to open widely due to trismus, which may preclude traditional intraoral radiographic techniques (Fig. 3.4). Occlusal films may identify palatal and mandibular or sublingual lesions (Fig. 3.5).

3.5.2 Computed Tomography

Computed tomography (CT) is a key modality for high resolution imaging of the hard and soft tissues of the head and neck. Given the expense and greater radiation exposure compared to plain films, CT should be ordered only when clinically warranted. CT can be particularly useful in determining the extent of a lesion prior to surgery, evaluating salivary gland pathology, assessing the status of cervical lymph nodes in cases of known or suspected malignancy, and evaluating deep neck space infections (Fig. 3.6). The need for an intravenous contrast agent

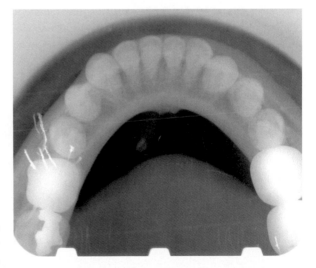

Fig. 3.5 Mandibular occlusal radiograph demonstrating presence of a salivary gland stone in the submandibular duct

should be determined in conjunction with the radiologist. Cone beam, or helical, CT for head and neck imaging provides high resolution images with significantly decreased radiation exposure compared to traditional CT (Fig. 3.7).

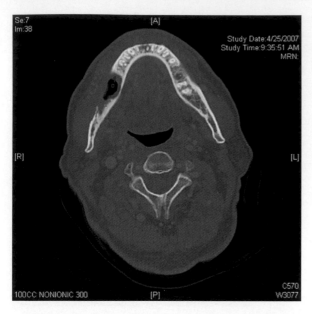

Fig. 3.6 Maxillofacial CT demonstrating extensive lytic changes in the right mandible secondary to osteoradionecrosis. High resolution CT imaging can delineate the location and extent of bone and soft tissue lesions more precisely than plain radiographs

3.5.3 Magnetic Resonance Imaging

While CT can be used for soft tissue imaging, magnetic resonance imaging (MRI) offers much higher resolution and provides greater ability to differentiate between different types of tissue. In addition MRI does not use ionizing radiation. MRI is primarily indicated for evaluation of salivary gland and other soft tissue lesions not readily visualized or palpable (Fig. 3.8). Despite an extensive body of literature, MRI has limited utility in the evaluation and diagnosis of patients with temporomandibular disorders. Overall, the clinical utility of MRI in oral medicine conditions is limited.

3.5.4 Other Imaging Studies

There are a number of additional imaging modalities that are not routinely used in the diagnosis of common oral medicine conditions. These include *positron emission tomography* (PET) scanning, which is used for diagnosis and surveillance of certain malignancies (Fig. 3.9); *ultrasonography*, which can be utilized for imaging of the salivary glands, thyroid, and cervical

lymph nodes; *sialography*, in which a radiopaque medium is injected into the salivary ducts to identify obstructive and degenerative changes (Fig. 3.10); and *scintigraphy*, which can be used to assess salivary gland function via radioisotope uptake. While not truly a diagnostic imaging modality, intraoral photography can be very useful for documenting mucosal lesions and evaluating changes over time (Fig. 3.11). This requires a specially equipped camera with proper illumination and focus adjustment, typically including a macro lens and ring flash (Fig. 3.12).

3.6 Cytology

Cytology specimens are quickly interpreted, and sampling is minimally invasive compared to traditional biopsy (Fig. 3.13). Interpretation requires an experienced cytologist, but can provide information about both infectious and noninfectious conditions of the oral cavity. Suspected *Candida* lesions are scraped with the intent of obtaining cellular material and smeared on a glass slide. They are then treated with potassium hydroxide, lactophenol blue, or other dye (or fixed and stained with Periodic Acid-Schiff), and analyzed under a microscope for the presence of characteristic fungal organisms (Fig. 3.14). Cytologic smears for HSV may reveal pathognomonic virally induced cellular changes such as multinucleated giant cells and "ballooning" cytoplasm (Fig. 3.15). Viral cytology is especially useful when culture results are inconclusive.

Enlarged lymph nodes, salivary gland masses, intrabony radiolucencies, and vascular appearing lesions may be initially evaluated using a fine needle aspiration biopsy technique (FNAB). This procedure must be performed by an experienced clinician and the specimen interpreted by an experienced cytologist, who should ideally be present at the time of the procedure (Fig. 3.16).

3.7 Tissue Biopsy

Tissue biopsy is the gold standard for definitive diagnosis of soft and hard tissue lesions. An *incisional* biopsy evaluates a small representative sample,

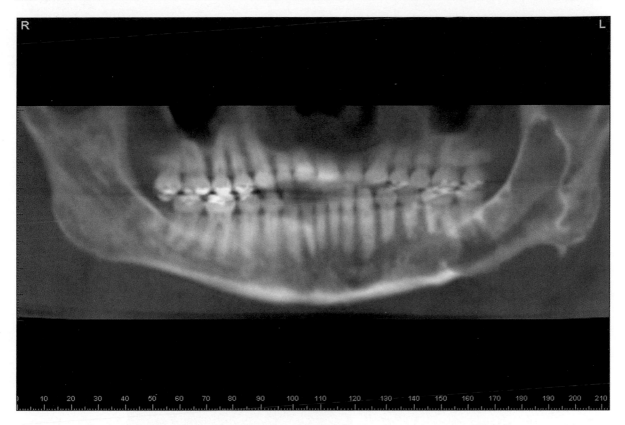

Fig. 3.7 Maxillofacial cone beam CT of the same patient in Fig. 3.4. While this panoramic reconstruction image offers little advantage over plain film panoramic tomography, the lesion can be evaluated in all planes

whereas an *excisional* biopsy involves removal and evaluation of the entire lesion. Biopsies may be submitted in formalin for routine histopathology or in saline or Michel's medium for direct immunofluorescence and other advanced studies (including tissue culture) that require nonfixed tissue. Immunohistochemical studies can be performed in many cases on both formalin fixed and fresh tissue samples and may be useful for determining or refining the diagnosis. The pathology laboratory should be consulted in advance when there are any questions as to how a specimen should be submitted.

The procedure in most cases is straightforward and often takes no more than 5 or 10 min to perform. Following informed consent, a small amount of local anesthetic with epinephrine (e.g., 1–2 cc of 2% lidocaine with 1:50,000 or 1:100,000 epinephrine) is injected, a 4.0-mm skin punch is rotated into the full thickness of the mucosa, and the specimen is grasped with tissue forceps and incised at its deepest point with scissors or scalpel (Figs. 3.17 and 3.18). In areas

where the tissue is closely attached to underlying bone, as seen on the hard palate and gingiva, a simple wedge biopsy with a scalpel is generally easier than using a skin punch. Small, well-defined lesions may be excised fully (Fig. 3.19). Placement of simple interrupted resorbable sutures or application of silver nitrate will effectively control bleeding following most incisional biopsies (Fig. 3.20). Pain following biopsy is typically mild, requiring only acetaminophen or ibuprofen in most cases; occasionally opiates are needed.

There are several important points to consider when performing a biopsy. If the lesion is nonhomogeneous, more than one area within the lesion should be sampled because early malignancies can present only focally in a field of dysplastic changes (Fig. 3.21). If the differential diagnosis includes a vesiculobullous disorder, the biopsy site should be perilesional, specifically avoiding any area of ulceration (Fig. 3.22). As ulcers lack epithelial layers, direct immunofluorescence testing cannot be ade-

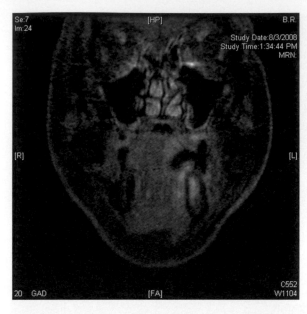

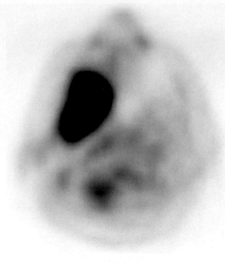

Fig. 3.9 PET scan demonstrating focal uptake in the right maxilla in a patient with recurrent non-Hodgkin lymphoma with intraoral soft tissue involvement. Diagnosis was confirmed with tissue biopsy

Fig. 3.8 Maxillofacial MRI demonstrating an aggressive inflammatory soft tissue lesion of the left lateral tongue

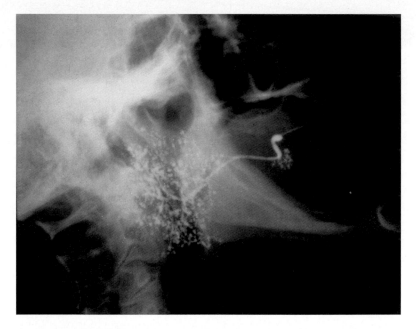

Fig. 3.10 Sialogram in a patient with Sjögren syndrome (see Chap. 8) demonstrating sialectasia secondary to chronic sialadenitis and fibrosis

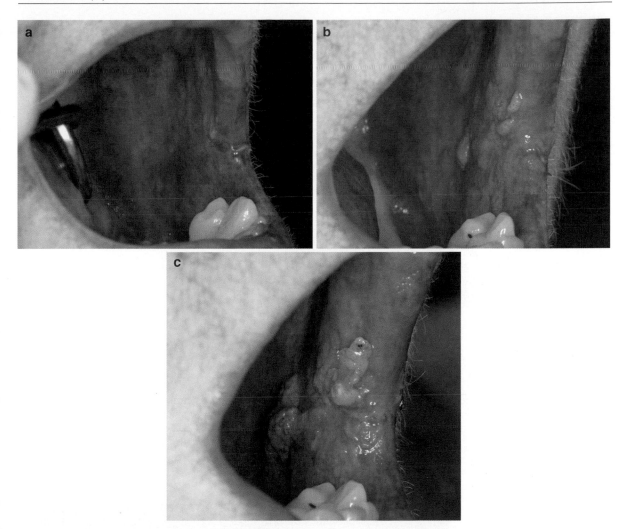

Fig. 3.11 Series of intraoral photographs of the left buccal mucosa in a patient with chronic graft-versus-host disease (cGVHD; see Chap. 11). (**a**) At initial presentation the patient reported intraoral sensitivity consistent with a long-standing history of oral cGVHD and was treated accordingly. (**b**) At 2-month follow-up multiple papillary growths were noted and biopsy was scheduled for 2 weeks later. (**c**) The patient returned 2 months after initial presentation, at which time the lesions had increased in size and biopsy confirmed invasive squamous cell carcinoma (see Chap. 9)

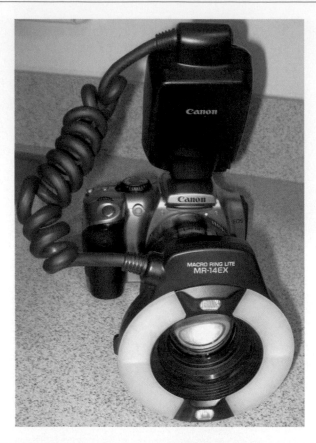

Fig. 3.12 Digital SLR camera equipped for intraoral photography with macro lens and ring flash

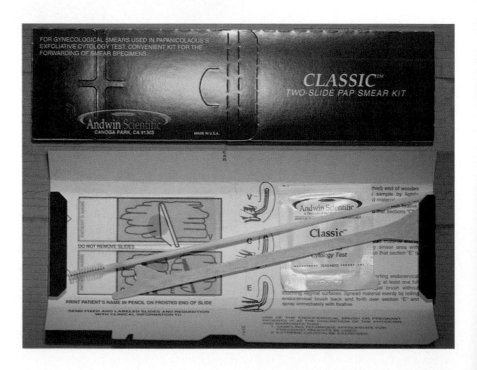

Fig. 3.13 Exfoliative cytology kit including glass slides, alcohol packet, wood spatula, and brush

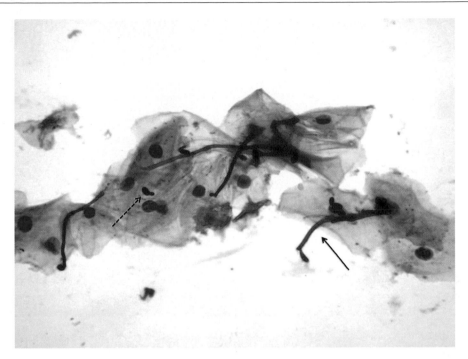

Fig. 3.14 Oral cytology specimen of a suspected fungal infection demonstrating *Candida* hyphae (linear organisms; *solid arrow*) and conidiae (ovoid budding organisms; *broken arrow*). Photomicrograph courtesy of Mark Lerman, DMD, Boston, MA

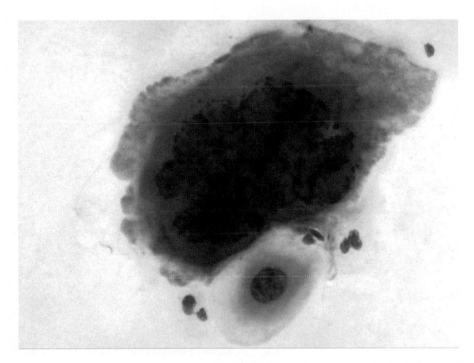

Fig. 3.15 Oral cytology specimen of a suspected herpes simplex virus infection demonstrating classic viral cytopathic changes in the cell above the normal keratinocyte. Photomicrograph courtesy of Mark Lerman, DMD, Boston, MA

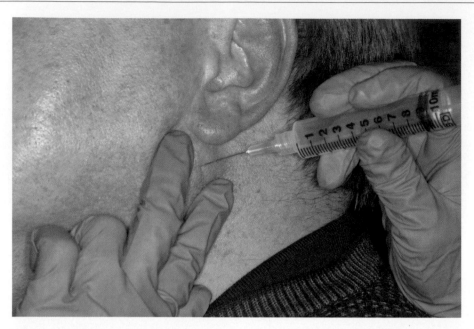

Fig. 3.16 Fine needle aspiration of an enlarged cervical lymph node. Photograph courtesy of Sook-Bin Woo, DMD, MMSc, Boston, MA

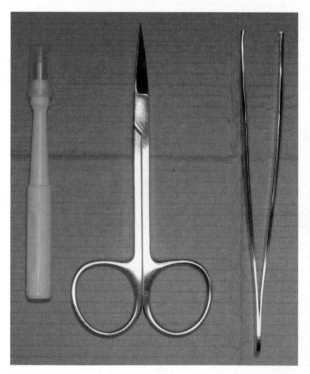

Fig. 3.17 Oral punch biopsy armamentarium that includes a 4.0-mm disposable punch, tissue forceps, and surgical scissors

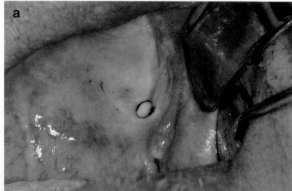

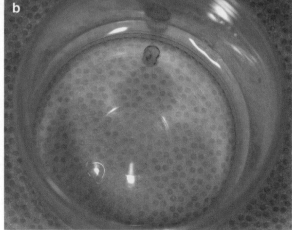

Fig. 3.18 Punch biopsy of an area of leukoplakia on the hard palate. (**a**) After rotation of the punch down to periosteum, prior to excision with forceps and scissors. (**b**) Excised surgical specimen placed in formalin

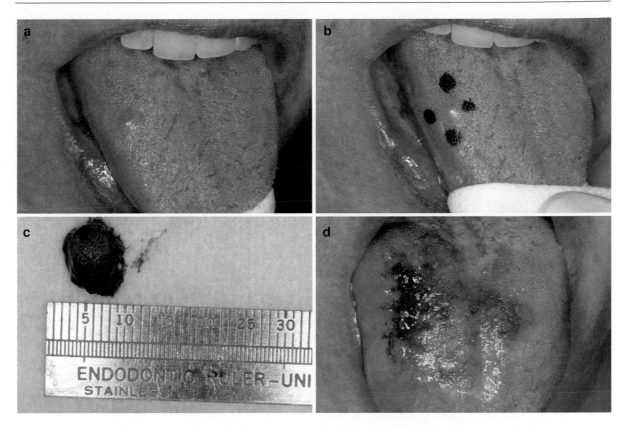

Fig. 3.19 (**a**) Excisional biopsy of a recurrent benign tongue neoplasm (spindle cell tumor). (**b**) Outline of excision marked with surgical pen to ensure adequate margins. (**c**) Gross pathology of excised specimen. (**d**) Postoperative sutured excision site

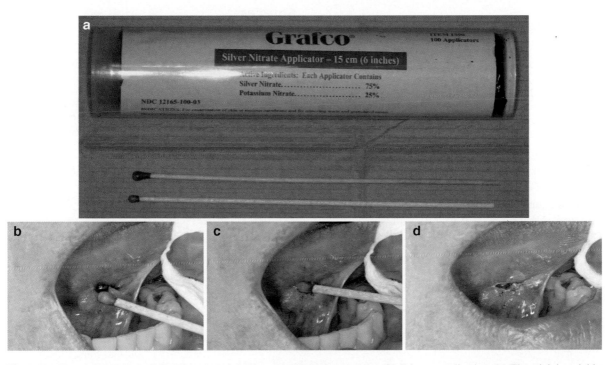

Fig. 3.20 Use of silver nitrate following a punch biopsy. (**a**) Silver nitrate sticks. (**b**) Prior to application. (**c**) The stick is quickly rotated and removed. (**d**) Biopsy site following application. The gray discoloration will gradually fade

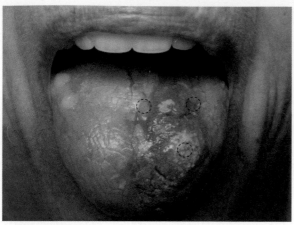

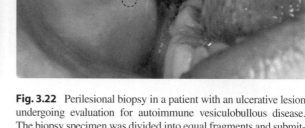

Fig. 3.21 Selection of multiple biopsy sites in a patient with a large area of erythroleukoplakia (see Chap. 9) to ensure adequate sampling

Fig. 3.22 Perilesional biopsy in a patient with an ulcerative lesion undergoing evaluation for autoimmune vesiculobullous disease. The biopsy specimen was divided into equal fragments and submitted for both routine histopathology and direct immunofluorescence

quately performed on specimens taken from such areas. All specimens should be carefully mapped and oriented. Regardless of the presumed clinical diagnosis, any tissue that is excised should be submitted for histopathological analysis. It is generally preferable to send specimens to a pathology laboratory with a board certified oral pathologist on staff or general pathologist with special training in oral pathology.

3.8   Adjuvant Tests

A number of commercially available adjuvant diagnostic tests and devices for the screening of premalignant and malignant lesions have recently been introduced to clinical practice. These include brush cytology (OralCDx Brush Biopsy, CDx Laboratories, Suffren, NY), toluidine blue vital tissue staining, tissue reflectance (ViziLite Plus, Zila Pharmaceuticals, Phoenix, AZ, and MicroLux DL, AdDent, Danbury, CT), and tissue fluorescence (VELscope, LED Dental Inc, Vancouver, Canada). There is considerable debate in the head and neck oncology, oral medicine, and oral pathology professional communities as to the value of these tests and devices, given that their

utility in aiding in the detection of oral cancer has yet to be definitively demonstrated. Of the above tests, toluidine blue may be useful in long-term surveillance of high-risk patients specifically as a tool to identify sites for biopsy.

Sources

Jordan RC, Daniels TE, Greenspan JS, et al. Advanced diagnostic methods in oral and maxillofacial pathology. Part 1: molecular methods. Oral Surg Oral Med Oral Pathol Oral Radiol Endod 2001;92:650–69

Jordan RC, Daniels TE, Greenspan JS, et al. Advanced diagnostic methods in oral and maxillofacial pathology. Part 2 : immunohistochemical and immunofluorescent methods. Oral Surg Oral Med Oral Pathol Oral Radiol Endod 2002;93:56–74

Lingen MW, Kalmar JR, et al. Critical evaluation of diagnostic aids for the detection of oral cancer. Oral Oncol 2008;44:10–22

Orel S, Sterrett G, Whitaker D. Fine Needle Aspiration Cytology, 4th ed. Elsevier, China 2005

Patton LL, Epstein JB, Kerr AR. Adjunctive techniques for oral cancer examination and lesion diagnosis: a systematic review of the literature. J Am Dent Assoc 2008;139:896–905

Shintaku W, Enciso R, Broussard J, Clark GT. Diagnostic imaging for chronic orofacial pain, maxillofacial osseous and soft tissue pathology and temporomandibular disorders. J Calif Dent Assoc 2006;34:633–44

Chapter 4
White Lesions

Summary The oral mucosa is normally semitranslucent, allowing the color of underlying tissues to show through to a variable degree. Lesions may appear white secondary to increased thickness of the epithelium or decreased submucosal vascularity, however, the etiology of white lesions is quite varied. This chapter reviews commonly seen white lesions of the oral cavity, with attention to differential diagnosis and treatment recommendations.

Keywords Hypertrophy • Hyperplasia • Keratin • Acanthosis • Hyperkeratosis • Leukoedema • Li nea alba • Lichen planus • Morsicatio • Leukoplaki a • Hairy tongue • Filiform papillae • Candidiasis • Oralhairyleukoplakia • Nicotinicstomatitis • Smoker's palate • Tobacco pouch keratosis • White sponge nevus • Exfoliative cheilitis • Angular cheilitis

4.1 Introduction

The oral mucosa is normally semitranslucent, allowing the color of underlying tissues such as fat, blood vessels, or melanin pigment to show through to a variable degree. This is affected by the thickness of the overlying tissue as well as the amount of surface keratin, concentration of submucosal fat or other substance, and density of the tissue capillary bed. For this reason, the thin nonkeratinized mucosa lining the vestibule and floor of mouth normally appears darker red than the thicker pale pink keratinized gingiva. Likewise, the vermilion zone of the lip appears red secondary to an abundant submucosal capillary blood supply.

Inflammatory conditions frequently result in increased redness (*erythema*) secondary to thinning of the mucosa and/or increased underlying vascularity.

Lesions most commonly appear white secondary to increased thickness of the epithelium, or to a lesser extent, decreased submucosal vascularity (Fig. 4.1). Thickening of the epithelium can be caused by epithelial hypertrophy or hyperplasia, edema, and increased production of surface keratin (*hyperkeratosis*). Thickening specifically in the spinous, or prickle, layer of the epithelium is referred to as *acanthosis*. Collapsed bullae or ulcerative lesions covered with a surface layer of fibrin may also appear white. Mechanical friction or other irritants to the mucosal lining can stimulate keratin production as a protective response. Some white lesions can be identified and treated on clinical grounds alone, whereas others require additional testing and/or biopsy for definitive diagnosis.

4.2 Leukoedema

This is a fairly common entity, seen as a generalized opacification or gray-white to milky opalescence of the buccal mucosa bilaterally (Fig. 4.2). It may appear filmy or wrinkled and cannot be rubbed off. The color becomes less evident or disappears entirely when the mucosa is stretched. It is usually noted as an incidental finding on exam and is asymptomatic; biopsy is not indicated. The etiology is not clearly established, however, there may be a hereditary component. This condition is more

J.M. Bruch and N.S. Treister, *Clinical Oral Medicine and Pathology*,
DOI 10.1007/978-1-60327-520-0_4, © Humana Press, a part of Springer Science+Business Media, LLC 2010

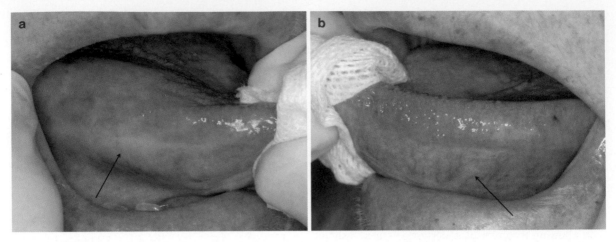

Fig. 4.1 Appearance of the ventrolateral tongue in a patient following radiation therapy. The right side (**a**), which was in the field of radiation, appears pale white with obliteration of vasculature. On the left side (**b**), which was not radiated, normal appearing vessels are easily visualized. Also note small petechia secondary to bite trauma

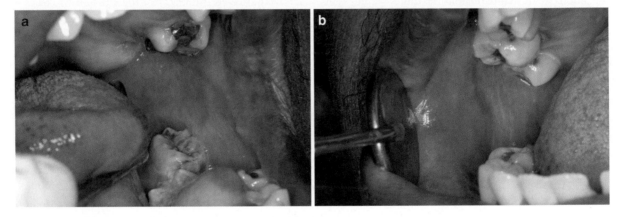

Fig. 4.2 Leukoedema of the (**a**) left buccal mucosa and (**b**) right buccal mucosa. The white changes disappear upon stretching of the tissue with a dental mirror

frequently seen in patients of African-American descent. Histologically, the tissue exhibits intracellular edema in the spinous cell layer of the epithelium. This is a benign condition, and no treatment is required.

Diagnostic tests: Stretching of the tissue with resulting diminished white color is diagnostic; no further testing is required.
Biopsy: No.
Treatment: None.
Follow-up: None.

4.3   Linea Alba

Literally meaning "white line," this is a focal hyperkeratosis resulting from chronic frictional trauma of the tissues rubbing against the adjacent teeth. It is most commonly seen as a horizontal white streak along the buccal mucosa at the level of the occlusal plane bilaterally and conforms to the configuration of the teeth in that area (Fig. 4.3). Frictional hyperkeratosis can also be seen focally in other commonly traumatized areas such as edentulous alveolar ridge spaces (Fig. 4.4), lips (Fig. 4.5), and lateral aspect of the tongue. This may be confused with lichen planus, which is a white lesion commonly occurring on the buccal mucosa (see Chap. 5).

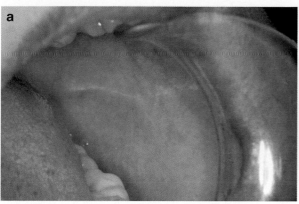
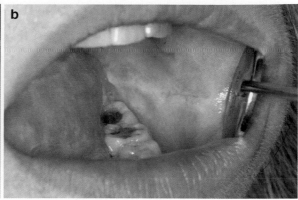

Fig. 4.3 Linea alba. (**a**) Fine, distinct linea alba of the left buccal mucosa. (**b**) Linea alba with a wide, shaggy appearance due to bite injury

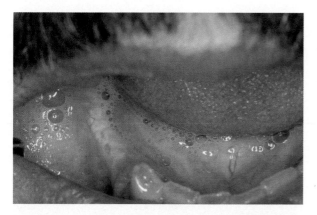

Fig. 4.4 Benign alveolar ridge keratosis. Frictional hyperkeratosis is common in edentulous areas

> **Diagnostic tests:** Diagnosis is based on clinical appearance.
> **Biopsy:** No, unless the appearance is atypical or diagnosis is uncertain.
> **Treatment:** None if classic linea alba is present on the bilateral buccal mucosa; otherwise attempt to identify and eliminate causative factor.
> **Follow-up:** None.

4.4 Cheek Biting

Hyperkeratosis from frictional trauma may be quite pronounced in cases of chronic cheek or lip biting or chewing (*morsicatio buccarum, morsicatio labiorum*). Lesions can appear ragged or frayed, with areas of ulceration or redness (Figs. 4.6–4.8). Chronic chewing

lesions of the tongue (*morsicatio linguarum*) can resemble *oral hairy leukoplakia*. The diagnosis is generally made on clinical grounds with biopsy performed if there is any doubt regarding etiology. It is almost always asymptomatic. There is no malignant potential and no specific treatment is required, other than an attempt to remove the source of irritation, after which the lesion should resolve in 1–3 weeks.

> **Diagnostic tests:** Generally none needed, as diagnosis is based on history and clinical appearance.
> **Biopsy:** No, unless the appearance is concerning for another diagnosis.
> **Treatment:** No specific treatment of the lesions is necessary. Patients should be made aware of the habit and encouraged to avoid chewing the tissues. Protective appliances can be fabricated if the problem is severe.
> **Follow-up:** None.

4.5 Hairy Tongue

Hairy tongue, or *lingua villosa*, is an entirely benign condition that can have a striking presentation. Elongation of the filiform papillae secondary to decrease in the desquamation of keratin can cause a white coating on the dorsum of the tongue, usually posteriorly (Fig. 4.9). The surface coating can become quite matted and hair-like, with gagging or sensation of irritation in some patients if the papillae become extremely long. Burning may be noted in cases of superimposed

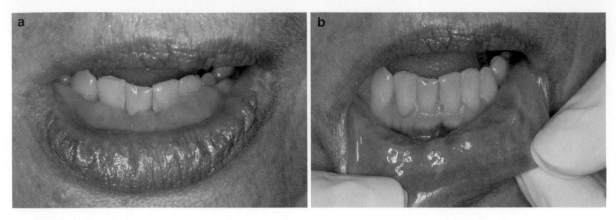

Fig. 4.5 Notably hyperplastic tissue of the (**a**) lower labial mucosa related to parafunctional activity; (**b**) with lower lip retracted

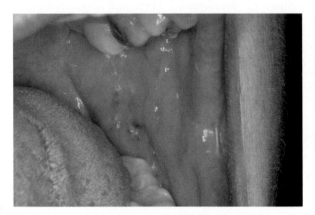

Fig. 4.6 Acute bite injury to the left buccal mucosa

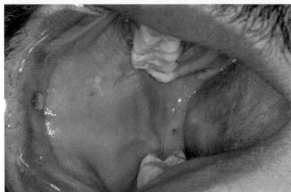

Fig. 4.8 Chronic bite injury to the right buccal mucosa. Parafunctional habits resulted in white lesions above the occlusal plane that could easily be mistaken for leukoplakia

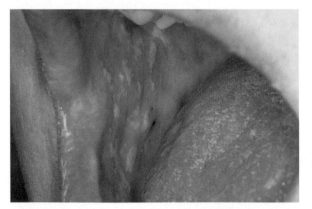

Fig. 4.7 Chronic bite trauma to the right buccal mucosa. The shaggy white tissue represents necrotic epithelial cells than can be easily scraped away without pain. A focal area of hemorrhage can be seen posteriorly

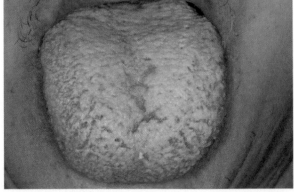

Fig. 4.9 Hairy tongue in a patient restricted to a soft diet

candidiasis (see Chap. 7). Trapping of chromogenic organisms and debris and staining from coffee or tobacco can cause a range of color variation from tan to black as well as pink or green (Fig. 4.10). The etiology is unclear, however, has been linked to use of antibiotics and certain mouthrinses, dehydration, xerostomia (Fig. 4.11), poor nutrition, and a soft or minimally abrasive diet (as may be seen in denture wearers). Treatment is generally not necessary, and elimination of any contributing factors typically results in complete resolution. If lesions persist and are bothersome to the patient, gentle brushing or scraping of the tongue can be recommended; trimming of the papillae may be necessary in extreme cases.

> **Diagnostic tests:** Diagnosis is based on clinical appearance. Identify causative or contributing factors.
> **Biopsy:** No.
> **Treatment:** Encourage well-balanced diet and smoking cessation. Gentle cleansing of the tongue can be helpful.
> **Follow-up:** None.

4.6 Oral Hairy Leukoplakia

This is a benign, well-demarcated, generally asymptomatic white lesion of the lateral tongue seen in HIV infected or immunosuppressed individuals. It can appear flat or raised, is often thick and corrugated, and frequently exhibits vertical ridge-like striations (Figs. 4.12 and 4.13). The lesions cannot be rubbed off, distinguishing the condition from *pseuodomembranous candidiasis* (see Chap. 7). OHL is believed to be associated with Epstein-Barr virus infection and is often seen as a precursor to development of an AIDS-defining illness. Malignant potential has not been demonstrated, and this is not considered precancerous.

> **Diagnostic tests:** None; diagnosis is usually established clinically in the context of HIV disease. Immune or HIV status should be ascertained if unknown.
> **Biopsy:** May be indicated to distinguish from *hyperplastic candidiasis* (**see Chap. 7**) or *leukoplakia* (**see Chap. 9**).
> **Treatment:** None.
> **Follow-up:** Observation.

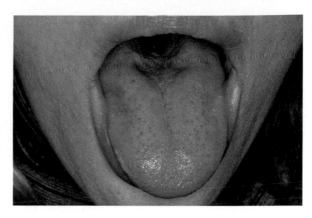

Fig. 4.10 Hairy tongue with yellowish orange pigmentation

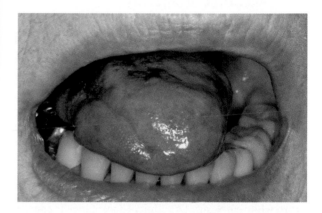

Fig. 4.11 Brownish colored hairy tongue in a patient with chronic atrophic glossitis following head and neck radiation therapy. Only the papillated regions of the tongue are affected

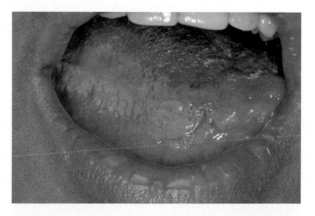

Fig. 4.12 Oral hairy leukoplakia of the right lateral tongue with diffuse white corrugated plaques. The patient also has a prominent hairy tongue, which is an unrelated finding

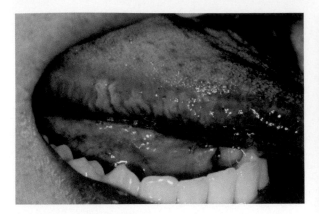

Fig. 4.13 Oral hairy leukoplakia of the right lateral tongue with focal linear white plaques

4.7 Nicotinic Stomatitis

Direct irritation of the palatal mucosa from hot tobacco smoke can lead to inflammatory changes which are initially erythematous, then become white secondary to progressive epithelial hyperplasia and hyperkeratosis. The palate exhibits a cracked or wrinkled appearance, with punctate red dots representing inflammation and squamous metaplasia of minor salivary gland duct orifices (Figs. 4.14 and 4.15). This is commonly referred to as smoker's palate. Any mucosa covered by a denture will be spared if the prosthesis is typically worn while smoking. The clinical appearance is usually diagnostic and biopsy is not necessary unless there are associated areas of ulceration or focal *erythroplakia* (see Chap. 9). This lesion is reversible with smoking cessation. Although the risk of malignant transforma-

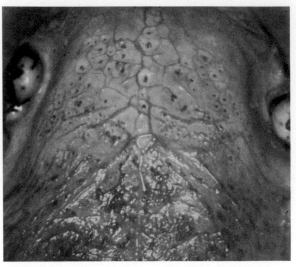

Fig. 4.15 Severe smoker's palate showing heavy keratinization and intensely inflamed duct orifices. Photograph courtesy of Ellen Eisenberg, DMD, Farmington, CT

tion is low and this is not considered a precancerous condition, its presence directly correlates with the intensity of smoking and is usually a marker of heavy tobacco use. Observation is therefore recommended in conjunction with careful screening of the entire oral cavity. Other white lesions related to tobacco are discussed in Chap. 9, including *leukoplakia* and *tobacco pouch keratosis*.

> **Diagnostic tests:** Diagnosis is based on clinical appearance.
> **Biopsy:** Generally not necessary unless lesions exhibit worrisome changes over time or persist after smoking is discontinued.
> **Treatment:** Smoking cessation.
> **Follow-up:** Observation.

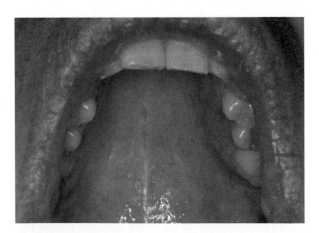

Fig. 4.14 Mild smoker's palate showing excessive keratinization of the hard palate and focally inflamed minor salivary gland duct orifices

4.8 White Sponge Nevus

This is a rare lesion, inherited as an autosomal dominant trait, which usually presents in childhood or adolescence without gender predilection. Genetic analysis has pinpointed the defect to genes encoding mucosal keratin (keratin 4 and 13). It appears as a thick corrugated or folded white plaque with a spongy texture that is typically located on the buccal mucosa bilaterally. It is generally asymptomatic and the clinical appearance is so distinctive that biopsy is not necessary. It can appear less frequently in other areas of the oral cavity as well as the esophagus, genitalia, and rectum, in which case biopsy may be needed. This is a benign condition and no treatment is required.

> **Diagnostic tests:** Diagnosis is made based on clinical appearance.
> **Biopsy:** No, unless appearance is not classic.
> **Treatment:** None.
> **Follow-up:** None.

4.9   Chemical Burn

A number of chemicals and medications can be extremely caustic to the oral mucosa if they come in direct contact. Inappropriate topical use of certain medications by the patient, such as aspirin tablets or powder held against the tissue, can result in significant trauma, causing coagulation necrosis and sloughing of the epithelium. Iatrogenic injuries can also be caused by agents such as sodium hypochlorite (a bleaching agent used for root canal irrigation), formocresol, silver nitrate, and acid etching solutions used during dental treatment. The initial lesion is usually white and leathery or wrinkled in appearance and generally very painful. If contact with the caustic substance was brief, which is usually the case, healing without scar or other complications should occur within 10–14 days and

palliative treatment with topical agents can be used. If more severe injury occurs, with surface desquamation and presence of deeper tissue necrosis, then treatment with antibiotics and debridement may be required. Over the counter alcohol-containing mouthrinses and other topical dentrifices may cause superficial chemical burns, including hydrogen peroxide in concentrations greater than 3% (Fig. 4.16). These are almost always painless and can be "peeled" away revealing normal appearing underlying mucosa.

> **Diagnostic tests:** Diagnosis is based on history and clinical appearance.
> **Biopsy:** No.
> **Treatment:** Palliative treatment with analgesics. Severe injuries may require antibiotics or tissue debridement.
> **Follow-up:** Until healed.

4.10   Exfoliative Cheilitis

This is an unusual chronic condition of the lips characterized by painful crusting and peeling of the superficial epithelium. In most cases the entire upper and lower lips are involved, and there may be associated erythema and swelling (Fig. 4.17). The cause is not firmly established, however, has been postulated to be secondary to repetitive lip irritation (such as chronic lip licking or picking), as well as other factitious or maladaptive behaviors. There may be an association with stress or depression in some patients. There is

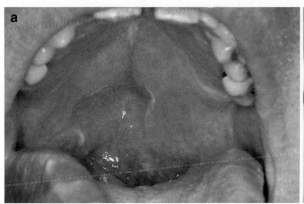 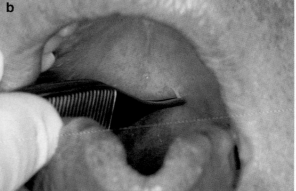

Fig. 4.16 Superficial chemical injury from use of an alcohol-containing mouthwash. (**a**) The palatal mucosa has a filmy appearance with areas that are peeling away. (**b**) The superficial necrotic layer can be painlessly removed with tissue forceps. Photograph courtesy of Sook-Bin Woo, DMD, MMSc, Boston, MA

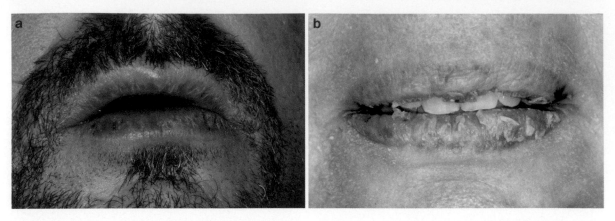

Fig. 4.17 Exfoliative cheilitis. (**a**) Mild case with crusting and peeling of the lips. (**b**) More severe case with extensive peeling and flaking

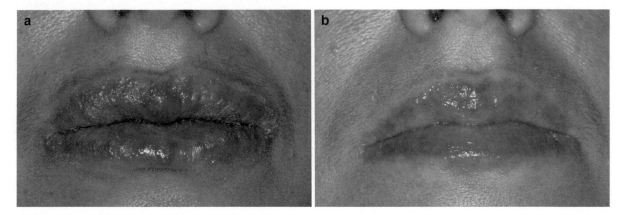

Fig. 4.18 Exfoliative cheilitis presenting with (**a**) raw and swollen lips with superficial crusting; (**b**) following several weeks of therapy with topical tacrolimus

rarely an infectious component, but secondary infection with candida should be considered if features consistent with *angular cheilitis* (see Chap. 7) are present.

> **Diagnostic tests:** None; diagnosis is based on clinical appearance and history.
> **Biopsy:** No.
> **Treatment:** Patient education regarding discontinuation of potentially causative habits or behaviors, such as lip licking. Use of topical petrolatum jelly usually results in resolution; tacrolimus 0.1% ointment once or twice daily may be effective in refractory cases exhibiting significant inflammation (Fig. 4.18).
> **Follow-up:** As needed while condition is active.

Sources

Chi AC, Lambert PR, Pan Y, et al. 2007 Is alveolar ridge keratosis a true leukoplakia?: a clinicopathologic comparison of 2,153 lesions. J Am Dent Assoc 138:641–51

Komatsu TL, Rivero ERC, et al. 2005 Epstein-Barr virus in oral hairy leukoplakia scrapes: identification by PCR. Braz Oral Res 19:317–21

Mani SA, Shareef BT. 2007 Exfoliative cheilitis: report of a case. J Can Dent Assoc 73:629–32

Martelli H, Pereira SM, Rocha TM, et al. 2007 White sponge nevus: report of a three-generation family. Oral Surg Oral Med Oral Pathol Oral Radiol Endod 103:43–7

Natarajan E, Woo SB. 2008 Benign alveolar ridge keratosis (oral lichen simplex chronicus): a distinct clinicopathologic entity. J Am Acad Dermatol 58:151–7

Woo SB, Lin D. 2009 Morsicatio mucosae oris: a chronic oral frictional keratosis, not a leukoplakia. J Oral Maxillofac Surg 67:140–6

Chapter 5
Immune-Mediated and Allergic Conditions

Summary A wide variety of immune-mediated conditions can affect the orofacial region. These range from localized immune responses, such as contact hypersensitivity, to systemic diseases with distinct and often prominent oral manifestations, such as the autoimmune vesiculobullous disorders. Oral lesions may precede the appearance of findings in other areas of the body or may represent the sole manifestation of the disease. Establishing the correct diagnosis is critical, as management strategies can vary considerably from one entity to the next. This chapter reviews the most commonly encountered immune-mediated conditions that have prominent oral manifestations, with specific guidelines for the use and interpretation of diagnostic tests and biopsy, and management strategies.

Keywords Angioedema • C1 esterase deficiency • ACE inhibitors • Orofacial granulomatosis • Melkersson-Rosenthal syndrome • Crohn disease • Ulcerative colitis • Inflammatory bowel disease • Sarcoidosis • Traumatic ulcerative granuloma • Aphthous stomatitis • Aphthous ulcer • Canker sore • Minor aphthous ulcer • Major aphthous ulcer • Herpetiform aphthous ulcer • Severe aphthous stomatitis • Behcet disease • Skin pathergy test • Erythema multiforme • Oral lichen planus • Lichen planus • Lichenoid hypersensitivity reaction • Desquamative gingivitis • Pemphigus vulgaris • Pemphigoid • Mucous membrane pemphigoid • Linear IgA disease • Nikolsky sign • Paraneoplastic pemphigus • Epidermolysis bullosa acquisita

as contact hypersensitivity, while others represent more widespread systemic disease with distinct oral manifestations, such as the group of autoimmune vesiculobullous disorders. The underlying pathobiological mechanisms are also quite varied and involve components of the innate and acquired immune systems. Some of these are very well characterized while others are not.

Determining the correct diagnosis is critical, as management strategies can vary considerably from one entity to the next. In some situations additional medical specialty consultation may be indicated, such as dermatology, ophthalmology, or otolaryngology. Oral lesions may precede the appearance of findings in other areas of the body or may represent the sole manifestation of the disease. This chapter is devoted to conditions in which oral findings are a primary feature. Systemic conditions that variably present with oral findings or complications are discussed in Chap. 11.

When evaluating a patient with a suspected immune-mediated or allergic oral disease that requires a tissue diagnosis, it is important to obtain a biopsy prior to initiating any topical or systemic immunosuppressive therapies, as these may mask characteristic or defining histopathological features. Since many of these conditions are chronic and require treatment with long-term topical and or systemic therapies, all patients should be followed on a regular basis. Detailed prescribing guidelines for the most commonly used medications are provided in Chap. 12.

5.1 Introduction

A wide variety of immune-mediated conditions can affect the orofacial region. Some present in a limited fashion secondary to a localized immune response, such

5.2 Angioedema

This is a condition characterized by rapid localized swelling of the skin or mucosa and underlying connective tissue. While angioedema can occur anywhere in the body, it most commonly presents in the head and neck region. The lips and tongue are most frequently affected; however, the floor of mouth and other areas of the face can also be involved. With involvement of the pharynx and larynx, patients may develop wheezing, voice change, and difficulty breathing; in severe cases this can progress to potentially fatal airway obstruction. The lower gastrointestinal tract can also be affected, resulting in symptoms including abdominal pain and diarrhea. Episodes typically develop within minutes to a few hours and resolve within 2–3 days, although changes can persist for as long as 1 week. Affected areas are characterized by painless, nonpitting edema with adjacent uninvolved tissues appearing completely normal (Fig. 5.1). Swollen tissues may be secondarily traumatized, but this is not a primary feature of the condition.

Angioedema occurs in hereditary and acquired forms. Hereditary cases typically present within the first or second decade of life and are caused by a deficiency in C1-esterase inhibitor, which is inherited in an autosomal dominant fashion. This results in uncontrolled activation of the complement cascade, causing tissue edema through mechanisms of vasodilation and increased vascular permeability. There is a rare form of acquired C1-esterase deficiency which is believed to be autoimmune in nature and is associated

in some cases with an underlying lymphoproliferative disorder. Nonhereditary angioedema may be medication induced, allergic, or idiopathic. The idiopathic variety is the most common of all types, affecting approximately 40% of patients with angioedema. The majority of medication-induced cases are caused by ACE inhibitors and these typically present within the first few weeks of therapy, although symptoms may occur years later. ACE inhibitors decrease the production of angiotensin II, a potent vasoconstrictor that is involved in the inactivation of bradykinin. Allergic cases are related to IgE-mediated mast cell degranulation with release of histamine, and symptoms typically develop within an hour of exposure. Common allergic triggers include nonsteroidal anti-inflammatory agents, opiates, other antihypertensive agents, contrast dyes, and foods (e.g., nuts, eggs, and shellfish). In some cases, stress and trauma have been implicated as triggers.

Oral lesions are usually self-limiting and resolve within 2–3 days. Patients with upper airway symptoms, including wheezing, gasping, or voice changes, should be evaluated emergently, as airway obstruction results in a significant risk of death in this condition. Patients with angioedema that is not obviously associated with an ACE inhibitor should be referred to an allergist or immunologist for comprehensive evaluation. Prophylactic therapies in patients with recurrent episodes include use of antihistamines (diphenhydramine, ranitidine); androgens (danazol, stanozolol), which directly increase levels of C1-esterase inhibitor; hemostatic agents (aminocaproic acid, tranexamic acid), which act through inhibition of plasmin; and glucocorticosteroids.

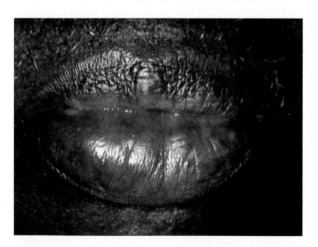

Fig. 5.1 Angioedema of the lower lip associated with ACE inhibitor use. The upper lip and facial skin are unaffected. Photograph courtesy of Andres Pinto, DMD, MPH, Philadelphia, PA.

Diagnostic tests: Patients should be referred to a specialist to further characterize the disorder and identify risk factors. Allergy and immunology work-up is generally indicated.

Biopsy: Not required in most cases.

Treatment: Androgens, hemostatic agents, antihistamines, and glucocorticosteroids can be effective prophylactic therapies.

Follow-up: Patients should be followed as needed to assess response to treatment.

5.3   Orofacial Granulomatosis

Orofacial granulomatosis (OFG) is a rare disease characterized by chronic recurrent painless swelling of the oral mucosa, lips, and perioral tissues (Fig. 5.2). The etiology is poorly understood, but in some cases can be attributed to hypersensitivity to certain foods or additives. The condition typically presents during early adulthood, and while generally asymptomatic, the disfiguring changes can have tremendous psychosocial consequences. Lesions are characterized by diffuse swelling, oftentimes with associated folded or fissured mucosal changes ("cobblestoning"), and focal areas of ulceration (Fig. 5.3). While the lips and perioral region are most frequently affected, any part of the mouth or face can be involved. OFG presenting with both

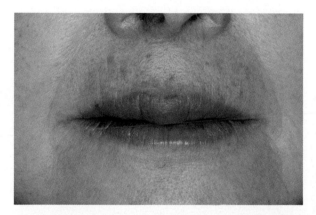

Fig. 5.2 Orofacial granulomatosis with prominent enlargement of the upper lip and characteristic vertical creases.

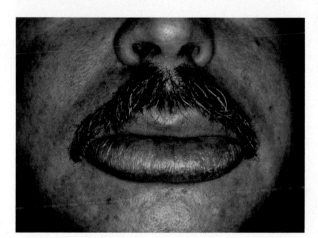

Fig. 5.3 Orofacial granulomatosis with painless swelling and fissuring of the lower lip. Photograph courtesy of Sook-Bin Woo, DMD, MMSc, Boston, MA.

fissured tongue and facial nerve paralysis is referred to as *Melkersson-Rosenthal Syndrome*.

The diagnosis of OFG is made based on biopsy of affected tissue. Histopathology demonstrates granulomatous inflammation and edema. A carefully recorded food diary may be helpful in identifying potential causative agents, but most cases are idiopathic. *Inflammatory bowel disease* (i.e., Crohn disease and ulcerative colitis) and sarcoidosis must also be considered, as each of these can present with similar clinical features (see Chap. 11).

Effective treatment of OFG can be challenging. If there are any suspected food triggers, these should be strictly eliminated from the diet. Episodes will generally respond to a short course of high-dose prednisone, which can be very effective in eliminating lesions in the short-term; however, this is not an appropriate treatment strategy for long-term management. Other medications that can be used include dapsone, hydroxychloroquine, sulfasalazine, minocycline, azathioprine, thalidomide, and anti-tumor necrosis factor (TNF-alpha) biological agents. For cases refractory to systemic therapies, intralesional corticosteroid therapy can be very effective. In many cases, intralesional injections must be administered regularly over an extended time period, even weekly, to maintain clinical remission.

> **Diagnostic tests:** None specific for OFG. Evaluate for sarcoidosis and inflammatory bowel disease.
>
> **Biopsy:** Yes, directly from the affected tissue.
>
> **Treatment:** Initial therapy consists of systemic and/or intralesional corticosteroid therapy. Preventive therapies include dapsone, hydroxychloroquine, minocycline, sulfasalazine, azathioprine, thalidomide, and anti-TNF-α biological agents.
>
> **Follow-up:** Patients should be followed regularly because even those receiving prophylactic therapy frequently develop breakthrough lesions.

5.4   Traumatic Ulcerative Granuloma

Traumatic ulcerative granuloma (TUG), sometimes also referred to as *traumatic ulcerative granuloma with stromal eosinophilia* (TUGSE), is a painful intraoral inflammatory lesion that is initiated by some type of traumatic event, most frequently a bite injury.

While the majority of traumatic injuries heal uneventfully in the oral cavity, TUGs transform into chronic, deep, and penetrating ulcerations that can be extremely painful (Fig. 5.4). The borders of the lesion appear

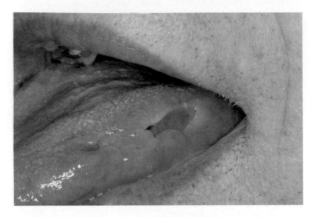

Fig. 5.4 Traumatic ulcerative granuloma of the left lateral tongue. There is a secondary, much smaller lesion anterior to the primary ulceration.

thickened and indurated with striations, representing an attempt by the surrounding tissue to heal. These can be easily mistaken for oral cancer clinically. There are no known risk factors, and these can be seen in any age group. The most common location for TUG is the posterior lateral tongue but lesions can also be seen in the buccal mucosa and soft palate (Fig. 5.5). Once established, TUGs rarely resolve without intervention.

Diagnosis requires an incisional biopsy, which should be taken from the ulcer margin to avoid obtaining necrotic tissue from the center of the lesion. In an otherwise healthy patient in whom infection (e.g., CMV, fungal) is not suspected, *squamous cell carcinoma* must be excluded (see Chap. 9). Histopathology demonstrates ulceration with a dense infiltrate of acute and chronic inflammatory cells including numerous eosinophils.

TUGs rarely heal spontaneously, and are typically present for several weeks before patients seek evaluation. Any obvious parafunctional habits or other factors contributing to persistent irritation, such as a fractured dental restoration, should be addressed and

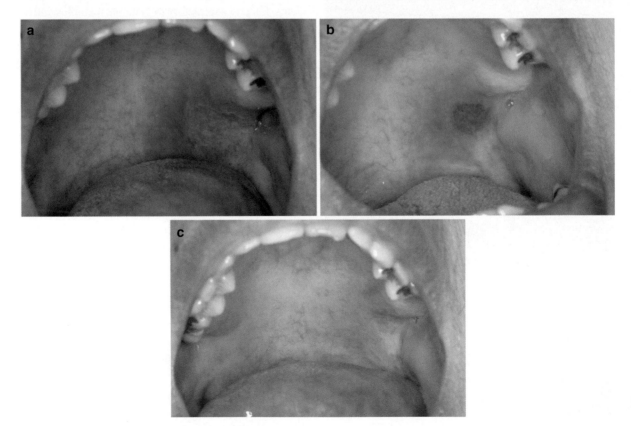

Fig. 5.5 Traumatic ulcerative granuloma of the left soft palate with extensive surrounding erythema. (**a**) This patient complained of severe odynophagia and referred pain to the ear. (**b**) Lesion 2 weeks, and (**c**) 4 weeks following combined intralesional and topical corticosteroid therapy.

corrected if possible. Once the diagnosis is made, the most effective first line therapy is intralesional corticosteroid injection (Fig. 5.5). This often requires multiple sequential injections on a weekly basis; at least three to four treatments should be provided before determining the lesion to be nonresponsive. A high potency topical corticosteroid gel, such as fluocinonide 0.05% or clobetasol 0.05% should also be prescribed and applied three to four times daily. Nonresponsive lesions can be treated with a 7–10-day course of high-dose prednisone. If still refractory, lesions should be considered for surgical excision; in some cases the inflammation is so deep and established that tissue debridement and primary wound closure is required, and referral to a specialist is recommended.

> **Diagnostic tests:** None; consider viral culture to rule out herpes simplex virus (HSV).
> **Biopsy:** Yes, to rule out other pathology including squamous cell carcinoma.
> **Treatment:** Topical and intralesional corticosteroid therapy.
> **Follow-up:** None following healing.

5.5 Aphthous Stomatitis

Recurrent aphthous stomatitis (RAS) is the most common painful oral mucosal disease, affecting approximately 20% of the population. Also referred to as *aphthous ulcers*, or the more commonly used lay term *canker sores*, RAS presents with a wide spectrum of severity ranging from a minor nuisance to complete debility. Characteristic oral ulcerations initially present in the first or second decade of life, making this one of the few immune-mediated inflammatory conditions seen in both children and adults. While the frequency of episodes often diminishes sharply during the third decade, patients are always at risk for developing recurrent lesions. Rarely, for reasons that are not understood, the frequency and severity of RAS can increase later in life.

Lesions appear clinically as nonspecific shallow round or oval ulcerations covered by a grayish-white fibrin pseudomembrane that is surrounded by a sharply defined erythematous halo (Fig. 5.6). Aphthous ulcers most commonly present as solitary lesions limited to the *nonkeratinized mucosa*, although exceptions exist and are discussed below. Ulcers may be preceded

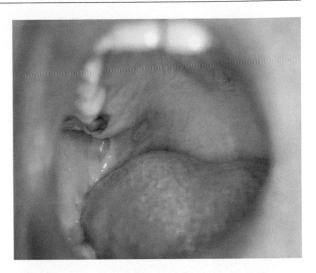

Fig. 5.6 Minor aphthous ulcer on the right soft palate with characteristic erythematous halo.

within hours by a tingling or burning sensation, allowing most patients to sense when they will develop a lesion. Once formed, ulcers typically last 7–10 days (with the first 3–4 days generally being the most symptomatic), and heal without complications.

The defining feature of RAS is pain. While lesions can be uncomfortable at rest, it is during function, such as speaking and eating, that symptoms are most intense. Like most painful oral inflammatory conditions, the location of lesions plays a major role in the severity of symptoms. Ulcers on the tongue can make speaking and chewing uncomfortable, while ulcers on the soft palate or in the esophagus can cause swallowing to be acutely painful. Ingestion of acidic foods and beverages can also be particularly uncomfortable.

There are four distinct clinical presentations: *minor, herpetiform, major and severe aphthous ulcers*. By far the most common, *minor aphthous* ulcers are less than 0.5 cm in diameter and follow the classic clinical pattern described above. An uncommon variant, *herpetiform aphthous ulcers* present as multiple small ulcerations that erupt in crops and subsequently coalesce to form an irregularly shaped lesion that mimics (but is unrelated to) those caused by HSV (Fig. 5.7; see Chap. 7). Although individual herpetiform aphthous lesions are less well defined and typically smaller in size than minor RAS lesions, the overall appearance is identical; these also typically heal within 7–10 days. *Major aphthous ulcers*, by definition larger than 1.0 cm in diameter, are seen far less frequently than minor lesions. These are deeper, more penetrating ulcers that can be intensely painful even at rest (Figs. 5.8–5.10). Major ulcers can last for weeks or months and may result in scar formation with resolution. *Severe aphthous stomatitis* is a clinical entity in which an affected individual is almost never without ulcers, resulting in debilitating chronic pain that can lead to weight loss, malnutrition, and considerable morbidity. Patients often suffer from multiple ulcers at any given time with new lesions developing as existing ones heal. The

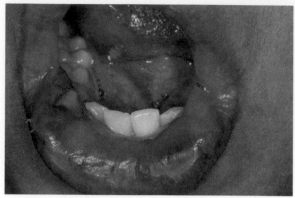

Fig. 5.9 Deeply penetrating major aphthous ulcer of the right lower lip. A second lesion can be seen on the tongue.

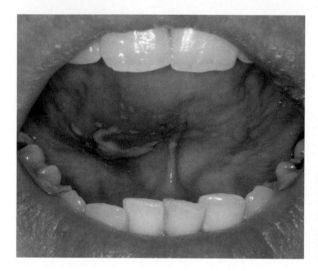

Fig. 5.7 Herpetiform aphthous ulcers of the ventral tongue. There is a central zone of coalescing ulceration with multiple crop-like smaller surrounding lesions.

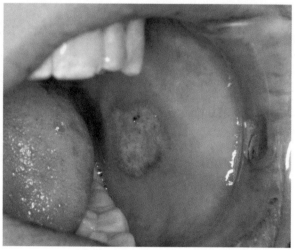

Fig. 5.10 Trauma-induced major aphthous ulcer of the left buccal mucosa. The patient accidentally bit both cheeks and subsequently developed bilateral major aphthae 2 days later. A focal area of petechiae shows where the bite injury initially occurred.

keratinized mucosa may also be affected in these patients (Figs. 5.11–5.14).

The etiology of RAS is poorly understood. Histopathology demonstrates nonspecific ulceration with a dense infiltration of acute and chronic inflammatory cells. T cells predominate and there are high local levels of the proinflammatory cytokine TNF-α. *Lesions are not contagious and are not caused by HSV.* Precipitating factors in some patients include stress, trauma, hormonal fluctuations, and certain foods and drinks. A number of conditions and diseases can

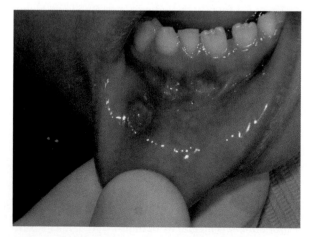

Fig. 5.8 Major aphthous ulcer of the right lower labial mucosa in a child exhibiting a wide margin of perilesional erythema.

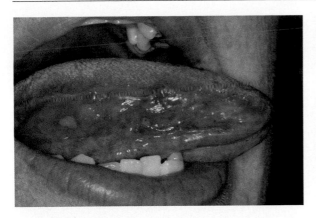

Fig. 5.11 Patient with severe recurrent aphthous ulcers with two minor ulcers of the right lateral tongue in addition to multiple other lesions throughout the oral cavity.

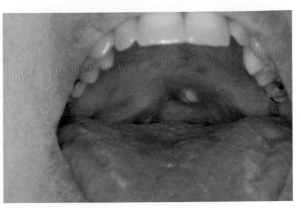

Fig. 5.14 Multiple soft palatal ulcerations in a patient with severe recurrent aphthous stomatitis. Due to the location of the lesions, all oral activities were very painful.

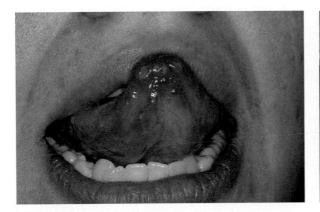

Fig. 5.12 Multiple minor aphthous ulcers of the tongue in a patient with severe recurrent aphthous stomatitis.

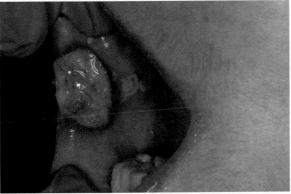

Fig. 5.15 Major aphthous ulcer of the anterior right buccal mucosa and commissure in a patient with advanced AIDS. Pseudomembranous candidiasis is also seen more posteriorly, although the two lesions are not specifically related (see Chap. 7).

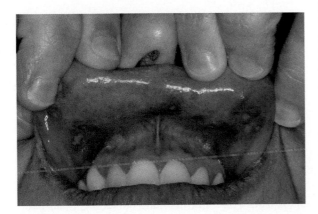

Fig. 5.13 Severe recurrent aphthous stomatitis with extensive ulcerations of the upper labial mucosa.

present with RAS, including deficiencies in folic acid, vitamin B12, and iron, inflammatory bowel disease (see Chap. 11), celiac disease, Behcet disease, and HIV disease. For reasons not well understood, patients with HIV disease can develop severe recurrent *major* ulcers that are often larger than 1.0 cm in diameter (Fig. 5.15; see Chap. 11).

Depending on the severity and frequency of outbreaks, management strategies range from simple palliative measures to systemic preventive therapies. The vast majority of patients with RAS never require any specific therapy, as their pain is tolerable and the diet may be modified as needed. Isolated painful episodes can be treated with over the counter products such as mucoadhesive agents and topical anesthetics. Topical

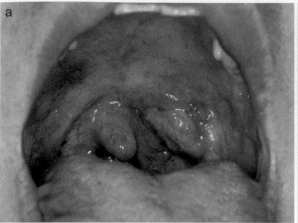 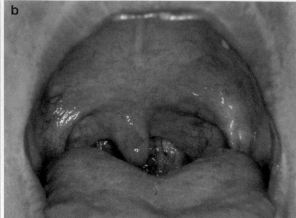

Fig. 5.16 Treatment of major aphthous ulcers with intralesional corticosteroid therapy. (**a**) Large, painful ulceration of the soft palate. (**b**) Same lesion 2 weeks following intralesional therapy with triamcinolone acetonide showing complete healing and resolution of symptoms.

application of high potency corticosteroid gels can significantly reduce sensitivity and may reduce healing time. *Major* lesions often require use of intralesional corticosteroids, however, may respond to intensive topical corticosteroid therapy (Fig. 5.16). For topical treatment of multiple or poorly accessible lesions, a corticosteroid rinse (e.g., dexamethasone 0.1 mg/mL) can be much easier to use and more effective than gels.

Patients with *severe* RAS often require systemic management. Acute painful ulcers are highly responsive to short courses of corticosteroids. Several agents can be effective in long-term prevention, including pentoxyfilline, colchicine, thalidomide, and azathioprine. Thalidomide is the only systemic agent that is FDA-approved for management of RAS, specifically in patients with HIV disease and major RAS. Topical corticosteroid rinses should also be included as part of any preventive approach. Patients responding favorably to treatment may cease developing ulcers altogether, or may experience lesions less frequently and of less severity. Even in patients who respond well to systemic steroid-sparing therapy, occasional short pulses of systemic corticosteroids may be necessary to control breakthrough symptoms.

Diagnostic tests: Blood test to evaluate iron, B12, and folate levels.
Biopsy: No.

Treatment: For occasional episodes: topical methylcellulose combined with benzocaine, viscous lidocaine, and high potency topical corticosteroids. For acute management of severe outbreaks: high-dose prednisone for 7–10 days. For prevention: pentoxyfilline, followed by addition of colchicine if adequate response is not achieved. Additional potentially effective agents include azathioprine and thalidomide.

Follow-up: All patients with *major* and *severe* RAS should be followed closely.

5.6 Behcet Disease

Behcet disease is a systemic disease with RAS as one of its defining features (Fig. 5.17). These include aphthous ulcers of the oral and anogenital mucosae, uveitis, inflammatory skin lesions, and other systemic findings such as arthritis, vasculitis, and CNS symptoms. Behcet disease is genetically determined and seen much more frequently in individuals from the Middle East and Far East. Systemic therapy is indicated in those with sufficiently severe clinical disease. In addition to the treatments for RAS discussed above, the use of anti-TNF-α biological agents, such as infliximab and etancercept, has demonstrated significant efficacy in patients with Behcet disease.

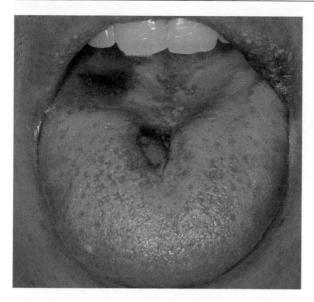

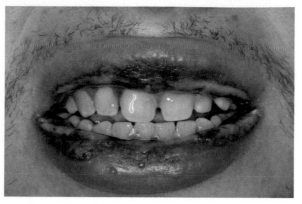

Fig. 5.18 Ulceration and crusting of the lips in a patient with erythema multiforme.

Fig. 5.17 Ulcerations of the tongue dorsum in a patient with Behcet disease. The patient also had painful genital ulcerations.

Diagnostic tests: Skin pathergy test in which the skin is penetrated with a sterile 20- to 22-gauge needle and evaluated 48 h later for an erythematous papule >2 mm.

Biopsy: Not required in most cases.

Treatment: Similar to treatment for RAS, including anti-TNF-α biological agents. Referral to an ophthalmologist for evaluation and management of ocular involvement.

Follow-up: All patients should be followed regularly.

5.7 Erythema Multiforme

Erythema multiforme (EM) is an acute, self-limiting mucocutaneous hypersensitivity reaction that presents with a wide range of clinical severity and appearance. Prodromal symptoms, including fever, malaise, and sore throat, are common and occur anywhere from days to 1–2 weeks prior to onset of lesions. EM can be divided into *minor* and *major* forms; *EM minor* is limited to skin, and *EM major* involves either the skin with at least one mucosal site or a single mucosal site with extensive involvement. *Stevens-Johnson syndrome* is a more severe manifestation of EM major in which there is extensive multisite involvement. Males are affected slightly more than females, with most patients presenting during their second or third decades of life. Recurrences are common.

Approximately 50% of cases of EM are associated with either medications or recent infection. The most commonly implicated medications include sulfonamides, nonsteroidal anti-inflammatory agents, and anticonvulsants. A careful medication history is therefore very important. A large proportion of cases are associated with either HSV or *mycoplasma* infection. In the case of HSV, EM most commonly occurs following outbreak of oral or genital herpetic lesions (see Chap. 7), but activation during subclinical shedding can also be seen. The subsequent lesions, however, are not HSV induced and do not show viral cytopathic changes. Approximately 50% of cases are idiopathic with no obvious cause.

Although not always present, the most consistent oral findings are crusting and ulceration of the lips (Figs. 5.18–5.20). Intraorally, lesions are characterized by nonspecific irregularly shaped ulcerations ranging from millimeters to centimeters in diameter with prominent surrounding erythema (Figs. 5.21 and 5.22). The keratinized mucosa is in large part spared, although the tongue dorsum may be affected, and lesions tend to occur toward the anterior aspect of the oral cavity. The genital and ophthalmic mucosa can also be affected. Skin lesions have a classic "targetoid" appearance (Fig. 5.23). Lesions develop over several days and can become intensely painful, resulting in inability to eat or speak (Fig. 5.24). The condition

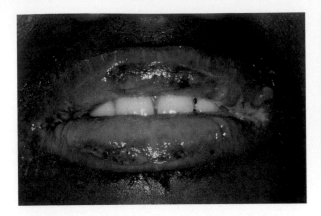

Fig. 5.19 Extensive ulceration of the lips in a patient with Stevens-Johnson syndrome. The patient had oral, ophthalmic, and genital ulcerations as well as skin lesions.

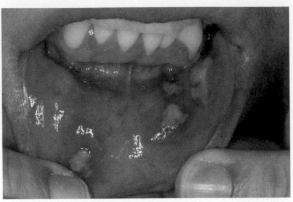

Fig. 5.22 Intraoral erythema multiforme in a patient with concurrent targetoid skin lesions. Although aphthous-like, the borders of the lesions are irregular and ragged in appearance.

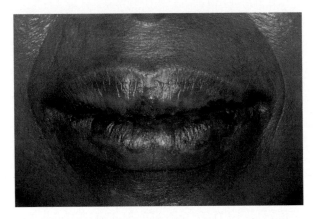

Fig. 5.20 Erythema and slight crusting of the lips in a patient with erythema multiforme. The patient had skin as well as oral lesions.

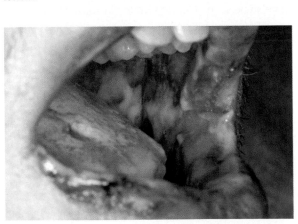

Fig. 5.21 Extensive intraoral ulcerations in a patient with erythema multiforme. The ulcers are irregular with extensive surrounding erythema. Given the severity of findings, this should be considered erythema multiforme *major* despite lesions being restricted to a single anatomic site.

is self-limiting, lasting anywhere from 2 to 4 weeks, and ulcerations heal without scarring (Fig. 5.25).

Diagnosis of oral EM is primarily clinical, although viral culture should be obtained and biopsy considered if the clinical presentation is atypical. A perilesional biopsy should be submitted for both histopathology and direct immunofluorescence (DIF). Characteristic findings include a high-density T cell infiltrate with prominent necrosis of the basal cell layer, subepithelial or intraepithelial blistering, and eosinophils. DIF studies are nonspecific but are helpful in ruling out other conditions such as *pemphigus* and *pemphigoid* (see below). When present, characteristic lip crusting and sparing of the keratinized mucosa easily distinguishes EM from primary HSV. When target lesions are also present, the diagnosis is very straightforward.

Treatment should be initiated as early as possible. The use of systemic corticosteroids in EM is controversial but is generally prescribed for patients with extensive oral involvement, and is given for 7–10 days without taper. Topical steroid rinses, three to four times daily, are also useful. Topical anesthetics, such as 2% viscous lidocaine, and systemic analgesics, including opiates, are usually necessary for pain management. Maintenance of hydration and nutrition is very important, especially in severe cases. For patients with a history of recurrent herpes labialis, appropriate antiviral therapy should also be prescribed.

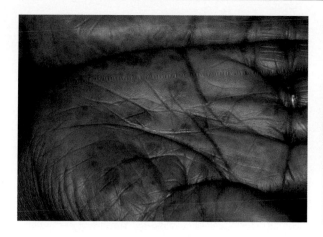

Fig. 5.23 Target lesions on the palms of the patient depicted in Fig. 5.20.

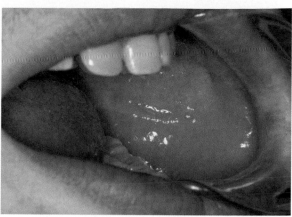

Fig. 5.25 The same patient in Fig. 5.24 after 1 week of high-dose prednisone therapy.

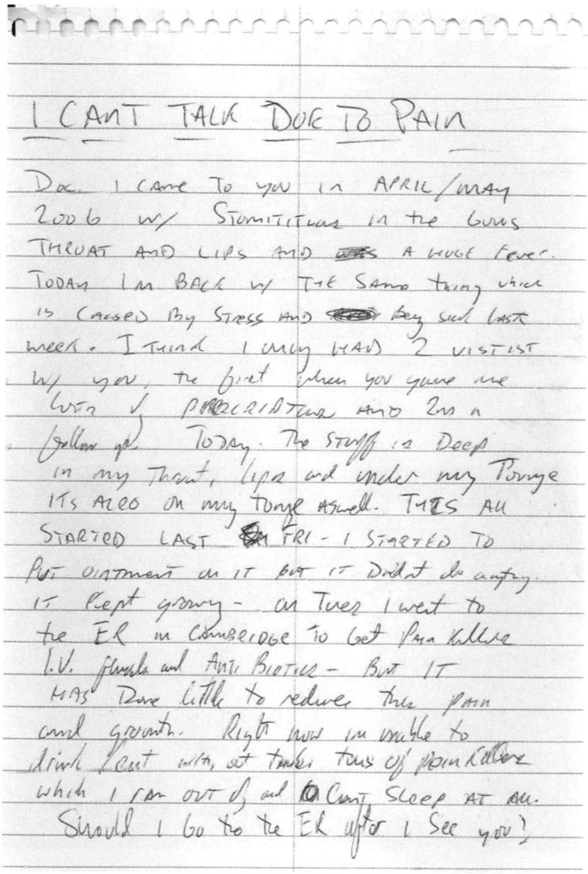

Diagnostic tests: Viral culture to rule out HSV.

Biopsy: Only if the clinical picture is not consistent with EM. Specimens should be perilesional and submitted for both routine histopathology and DIF to rule out autoimmune vesiculobullous disorders.

Treatment: Systemic and topical corticosteroids for severe cases; topical corticosteroids alone for milder cases. Pain management and nutritional support.

Follow-up: Patients should be reevaluated 1 week after initiating therapy. For patients with a history of recurrent HSV and recurrent EM, long-term prophylaxis with acyclovir or valacyclovir should be initiated.

Fig. 5.24 The patient in Fig. 5.21 was in so much pain that he was not able to speak or eat.

5.8   Oral Lichen Planus (OLP)

Lichen planus is a chronic mucocutaneous T cell-mediated inflammatory condition that affects nearly 1% of the adult population. Oral lesions are common and may be the only manifestation of disease in many cases. Although the extent and severity of lesions may fluctuate over time, the condition tends to be persistent once established. Women are affected slightly more than men, with most patients diagnosed during their fourth through seventh decades of life. Since lichen planus can affect the skin as well as other mucosal sites including the larynx and genitalia, patients should be specifically questioned regarding extra-oral symptoms.

OLP most likely represent a heterogeneous group of hypersensitivity reactions exhibiting indistinguishable clinical and histopathological features. If a specific causative agent, typically a medication, is identified, the condition may be referred to as a *lichenoid hypersensitivity reaction*. Numerous medications have been associated with OLP including antihypertensive and nonsteroidal anti-inflammatory agents. Discontinuation of the suspected trigger may be effective, although cross-sensitivity with other medications is common and lesions may persist. Amalgam dental restorations (silver fillings) and cinnamon flavored products have been associated with localized *contact lichenoid hypersensitivity reactions*. These lesions appear clinically identical to OLP, occur at the site of contact with the offending agent, and generally resolve following removal of the causative agent. The majority of cases of OLP are idiopathic with no obvious cause.

Patients may complain of symptoms, which are highly variable, but often consist of oral sensitivity to toothpaste, acidic substances, alcohol, carbonated beverages, spicy or salty foods, and abrasive foods. The majority of patients, even those with extensive mucosal involvement, are otherwise typically symptom-free.

There are three distinct clinical presentations of OLP, any of which may be observed in an affected individual at a given time: *reticular, erythematous,* and *erosive. Reticular* lesions, also known as *Wickham's striae*, appear as lacey white mucosal changes due to a focal pattern of hyperkeratosis. This is a classic distinctive feature of OLP that is also seen in skin lesions (Figs. 5.26–5.28). A less common variation of the reticular form includes *plaque-like* changes (Fig. 5.29), which may be difficult to differentiate from true leukoplakia (see Chap. 9). *Erythematous* lesions, which are often intimately associated with reticular changes, are due to thinning or atrophy of the epithelium with inflammation of the underlying connective tissue (Fig. 5.30). *Erosive/ Ulcerative OLP* is the most severe form, and is almost always associated with reticular and erythematous changes (Figs. 5.31–5.33). Patients with extensive ulcerative lesions tend to have more severe symptoms than those with purely reticular changes, although even patients with apparently "mild" clinical disease may experience significant morbidity.

Any intraoral site can be affected, with the most common being the buccal mucosa and lateral tongue; these lesions are almost always present bilaterally. The

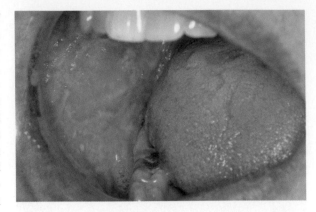

Fig. 5.26 Oral lichen planus of the right buccal mucosa exhibiting a fine reticular pattern and minimal erythema.

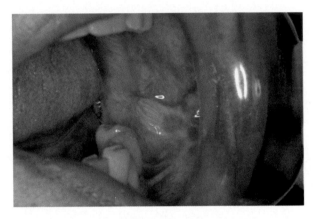

Fig. 5.27 Oral lichen planus of the left buccal mucosa with prominent linear reticulation and erythema.

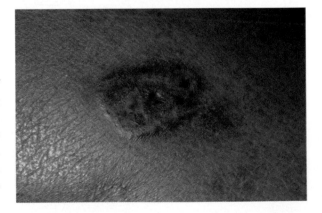

Fig. 5.28 Lichen planus of the skin in an African-American patient with concurrent oral lesions. The same characteristic reticulation seen in the mouth can be seen with skin lesions.

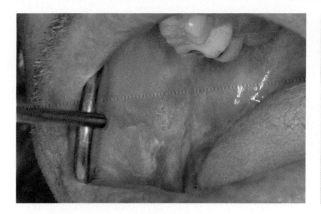

Fig. 5.29 Plaque-like oral lichen planus of the right buccal mucosa. While some areas of reticulation can be seen, these lesions are characterized by white plaques that can easily be mistaken for leukoplakia. There are also focal areas of ulceration.

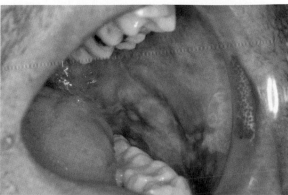

Fig. 5.31 Oral lichen planus of the left buccal mucosa with reticulation, erythema, and focal ulcerations.

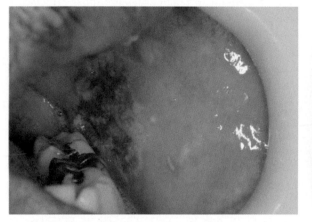

Fig. 5.30 Oral lichen planus of the left buccal mucosa with reticulation and severe erythema.

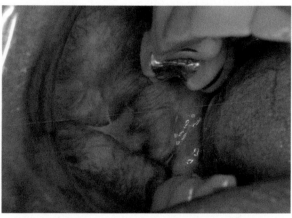

Fig. 5.32 Oral lichen planus of the right buccal mucosa with prominent reticulation, erythema, and central ulceration.

gingiva and alveolar mucosa are also relatively common areas (Figs. 5.34–5.36); if this represents the only site of involvement, and erythema and/or ulceration are present, the clinical condition is called *desquamative gingivitis*. Fifty percent of cases of desquamative gingivitis ultimately prove to be *mucous membrane pemphigoid (MMP)*, 25% are OLP, and the remaining 25% are composed of other vesiculobullous disorders including *pemphigus vulgaris* and *linear IgA disease* (see below). The extent and severity of lesions can fluctuate over time and are often exacerbated during periods of illness and stress.

In patients presenting with classic appearing bilateral reticulated lesions of the buccal mucosa, the diagnosis can be made by clinical examination alone. A biopsy should be obtained, avoiding ulcerative areas due to lack

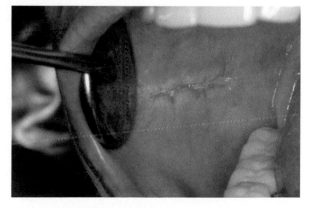

Fig. 5.33 Oral lichen planus of the right buccal mucosa with focal linear ulceration.

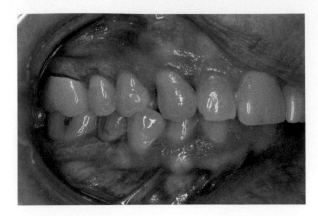

Fig. 5.34 Oral lichen planus with prominent reticulation restricted to the gingiva.

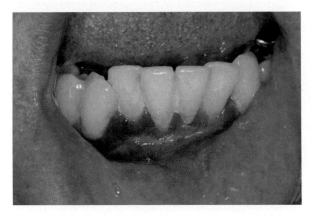

Fig. 5.35 Oral lichen planus presenting with only desquamative gingivitis. Without prominent visible reticulation, biopsy is needed for diagnosis.

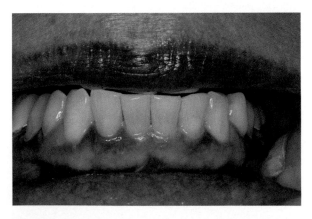

Fig. 5.36 Oral lichen planus with erythema and reticulation of the anterior mandibular gingiva.

of intact epithelium, if the diagnosis is not evident. In the case of desquamative gingivitis, the specimen should be submitted for both routine histopathology as well as DIF. Histopathological features of reticulated lesions include hyperkeratosis, a "saw-toothed" appearance of the epithelial rete ridges, band-like lymphocytic (primarily T-cell) infiltrate in the connective tissue just below the basement membrane, and basal cell degeneration. There are no blood tests that help with the diagnosis of OLP.

Treatment should be dictated by the severity of symptoms rather than clinical appearance. Patients with asymptomatic OLP do not require treatment; in symptomatic cases the mainstay of therapy is high potency topical corticosteroids. Limited lesions are treated with a topical gel; more extensive or difficult to reach areas are most effectively treated with a rinse. Patients with desquamative gingivitis benefit from custom fabricated trays to apply the medication.

In refractory cases, topical tacrolimus is used in addition to corticosteroids. This is commercially available as an ointment, but can be formulated as a rinse by a compounding pharmacy. While topical therapies are very safe and can be used long term, they should be applied as infrequently as possible, balancing the need to provide adequate control of symptoms with the ability to intensify therapy in the event of clinical flares.

In cases where topical therapy is inadequate, a short course of high-dose prednisone can be effective for severe flares. Nonsteroidal systemic therapies include hydroxychloroquine, azathioprine, cyclosporine, tacrolimus, and thalidomide, and in severe refractory cases, extracorporeal photopheresis can be considered. Due to the lack of adequate controlled trials of systemic agents for OLP, there is little evidence to recommend the use of one over another. Once the disease is under good control, attempts should be made to taper any systemic agents to the lowest effective dose possible while maximizing the effects of topical treatment.

The most serious complication of OLP is malignant transformation to squamous cell carcinoma (see Chap. 9). It is estimated that approximately 1% of cases of OLP ultimately develop into oral cancer. The epidemiology and risk factors are poorly characterized, but it is generally thought that the more severe or refractory cases represent the highest risk. For this reason, any suspicious changes should be biopsied and all patients with OLP should be seen at least annually.

Diagnostic tests: None.

Biopsy: Only when clinical presentation is not classic (reticular) in appearance.

Treatment: Topical corticosteroids and topical tacrolimus are the mainstay of therapy. When necessary, systemic agents should be considered. For severe refractory cases consider extracorporeal photopheresis or anti-TNF-α biological therapy.

Follow-up: Patients should be followed carefully to evaluate response to therapy. Stable or asymptomatic cases should be followed annually; assess carefully for malignancy.

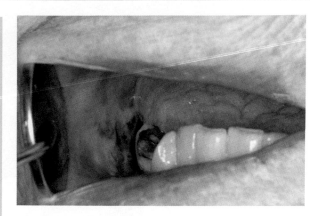

Fig. 5.37 Mucous membrane pemphigoid with nonspecific ulceration of the posterior right buccal mucosa.

5.9 Mucous Membrane Pemphigoid

While there are several variants of pemphigoid, MMP most commonly affects the oral mucosa. MMP is an autoimmune vesiculobullous blistering disease characterized by autoreactive antibodies that target the hemidesmosomal complex of the epithelial basement membrane, resulting in subepithelial tissue separation. This disease most frequently presents during the fifth to seventh decades of life and affects women at nearly twice the rate of men. Aside from pain, one of the greatest complications of MMP is scarring, which can lead to blindness in the setting of ocular lesions. When disease manifestations are limited to the oral mucosa, scarring is exceedingly rare. All patients should be questioned about extraoral symptoms including involvement of the throat, nose, eyes, and genitals.

Any oral mucosal site can be affected. Intact blisters may be observed, however, these generally rupture quickly and leave irregularly shaped ulcerations (Fig. 5.37). Many patients present only with desquamative gingivitis (Fig. 5.38). Diagnosis of MMP relies on perilesional biopsy submitted for both histopathology and DIF studies. Histopathology demonstrates clear subepithelial clefting (Fig. 5.39). DIF shows distinct deposition of IgG and complement at the basement membrane (Fig. 5.40). Indirect immunofluorescence results are variable.

If lesions are not limited to the oral mucosa, systemic therapy with corticosteroids and steroid-sparing agents is generally indicated. Purely oral cases of MMP should be treated based on symptoms and generally respond well to topical corticosteroids or tacrolimus. Desquamative gingivitis is most effectively

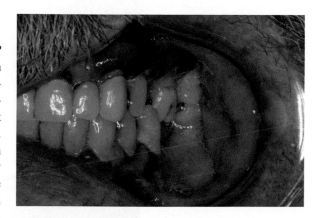

Fig. 5.38 Mucous membrane pemphigoid presenting as desquamative gingivitis. The gingiva is erythematous with a focal area of ulceration on the interdental papilla between the mandibular canine and premolar.

treated with custom trays containing high potency corticosteroid gels (Fig. 5.41).

Diagnostic tests: None.

Biopsy: Yes; the specimen should be taken from a perilesional area and submitted for both routine histopathology and DIF.

Treatment: Topical corticosteroids (first-line) or tacrolimus (second-line) as the mainstay of therapy. Systemic agents if refractory: prednisone, mycophenolate mofetil, azathioprine, dapsone, cyclosporine, and tacrolimus. For severe refractory cases consider rituximab, IVIG, and extracorporeal photopheresis.

Follow-up: Patients should be followed carefully while evaluating response to therapy. Patients with stable disease should be followed at least annually.

Fig. 5.39 Mucous membrane pemphigoid histopathology (H&E stain) demonstrating a clear subepithelial separation at the basement membrane. Photomicrograph courtesy of Mark Lerman, DMD, Boston, MA.

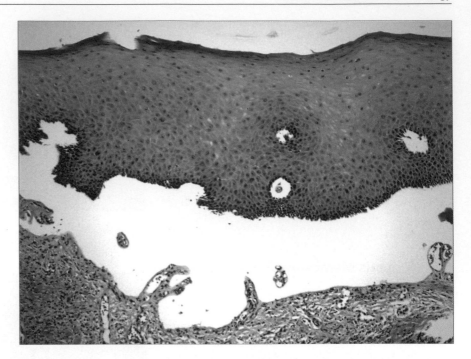

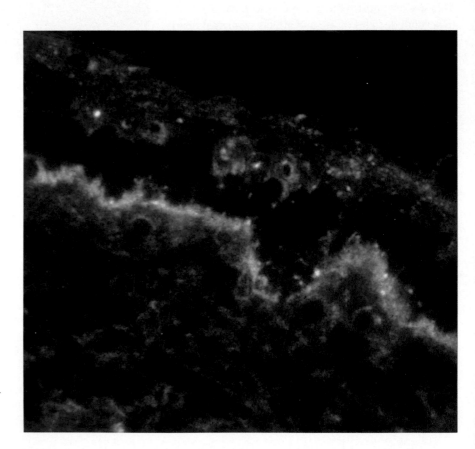

Fig. 5.40 Mucous membrane pemphigoid (direct immuno-fluorescence) showing a prominent band of reactivity along the basement membrane. Photomicrograph courtesy of Stephen Sonis, DMD, DMSc, Boston, MA.

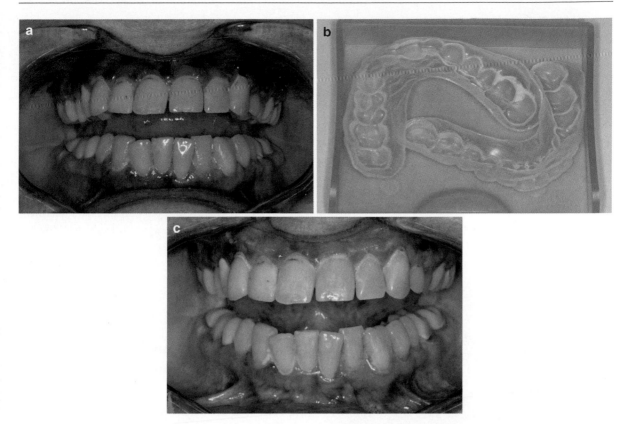

Fig. 5.41 Soft trays for localized intensive application of topical therapy for desquamative gingivitis. (**a**) Patient with extensive desquamative gingivitis due to mucous membrane pemphigoid. (**b**) Soft trays were made and the patient was instructed to treat with fluocinonide gel 0.05% daily. (**c**) After 1 month of therapy with almost complete resolution of all signs and symptoms.

5.10 Pemphigus Vulgaris

The term "pemphigus" encompasses a group of autoimmune vesiculobullous blistering diseases, the most common of which is *pemphigus vulgaris*. Although this variant is still potentially severe, it is no longer the life-threatening condition it was prior to the introduction of corticosteroids. Circulating IgG autoantibodies target the desmosomal complex, specifically binding the surface glycoproteins desmoglein 1 and 3, resulting in intraepithelial splitting. Females are affected slightly more frequently than males, with most patients presenting during the fourth to sixth decades of life. Patients of Mediterranean and Ashkenazi Jewish descent are affected at a higher rate. The skin is almost always involved; however, the appearance of oral lesions usually precedes cutaneous manifestations. Other mucosal sites, such as the nasal and anogenital regions, may be involved.

Oral lesions appear as well-demarcated, irregular erythematous erosions and ulcerations that can become quite large and very painful (Figs. 5.42 and 5.43). Commonly affected oral sites are the buccal mucosa, palate, and gingiva. Intact bullae are rarely observed. A *positive Nikolsky sign* is a nonspecific feature in which a blister may be induced by rubbing unaffected skin or mucosa; this may be seen in pemphigus vulgaris but also in MMP or various other conditions. As any other mucosal site can be affected, patients should be questioned regarding extraoral symptoms and referred to an appropriate specialist as necessary. Without intervention, lesions tend to persist for weeks to months, often continuing to grow in size.

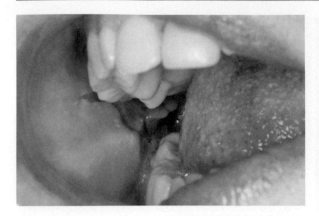

Fig. 5.42 Pemphigus vulgaris with well-defined ulceration and normal appearing surrounding tissue.

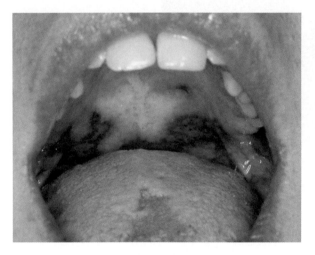

Fig. 5.43 Palatal lesions in a patient with pemphigus vulgaris.

Diagnosis requires a perilesional tissue biopsy submitted for both histopathology and DIF studies. Histopathological findings include intraepithelial separation, typically just above the basal cell layer, and *acantholysis*, or separation of the epithelial cells from each other (Fig. 5.44). DIF demonstrates a classic intercellular binding pattern of IgG (Fig. 5.45). Indirect immunofluorescence (IIF) studies are typically positive for antibodies against desmosomal glycoproteins.

Management of pemphigus vulgaris invariably requires systemic therapy. Corticosteroids and steroid-sparing immunomodulatory agents (azathioprine, cyclosporine, tacrolimus, and mycophenolate mofetil) are the mainstays of treatment. Breakthrough lesions are common, in which case topical corticosteroids

play an important role. Truly refractory cases of pemphigus vulgaris may be controlled with intravenous immunoglobulin therapy, rituximab, and extracorporeal photopheresis.

> **Diagnostic tests:** IIF is generally positive.
> **Biopsy:** Yes, perilesional and submitted for both routine histopathology and DIF.
> **Treatment:** Topical corticosteroids, or if ineffective, topical tacrolimus for oral lesions. Systemic agents include prednisone, mycophenolate mofetil, azathioprine, dapsone, cyclosporine, and tacrolimus. For severe refractory cases consider rituximab, IVIG, and extracorporeal photopheresis.
> **Follow-up:** Patients should be followed carefully while evaluating response to therapy. Patients with stable disease should be followed at least annually.

5.11 Other Autoimmune Vesiculobullous Diseases

5.11.1 Paraneoplastic Pemphigus

A very rare but important variant of pemphigus vulgaris seen exclusively in patients with underlying neoplasia is termed *paraneoplasic pemphigus*. This condition has been associated with non-Hodgkin lymphoma, chronic lymphocytic leukemia, sarcomas, thymomas, and Castleman disease. Circulating autoantibodies are produced that target desmosomes and hemidesmosomes, resulting in potentially severe skin and mucosal lesions. Diagnosis and management of the underlying neoplasm are essential and generally results in resolution of the mucocutaneous disease.

5.11.2 Epidermolysis Bullosa Acquisita

Epidermolysis bullosa is a rare chronic autoimmune subepidermal vesiculobullous disorder that affects the skin and mucosa. Onset is very early in life, however, severity varies greatly such that milder forms of the disease are often not identified for many years. Autoantibodies target multiple hemidesmosomal antigens, in particular components of type VII collagen,

Fig. 5.44 Pemphigus vulgaris histopathology (H&E stain) demonstrating suprabasilar separation of cells and individual acantholytic (Tzanck) cells within the cleft (*black arrow*). Photomicrograph courtesy of Mark Lerman, DMD, Boston, MA.

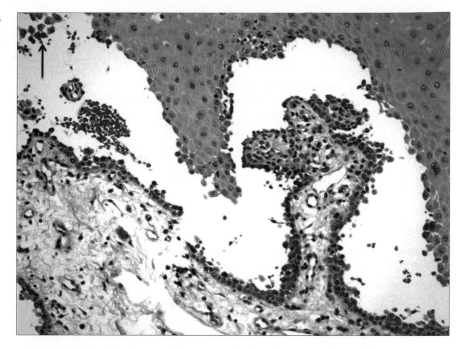

Fig. 5.45 Pemphigus vulgaris (direct immunofluorescence) showing prominent reactivity between keratinocytes throughout the epithelium. Photomicrograph courtesy of Stephen Sonis, DMD, DMSc, Boston, MA.

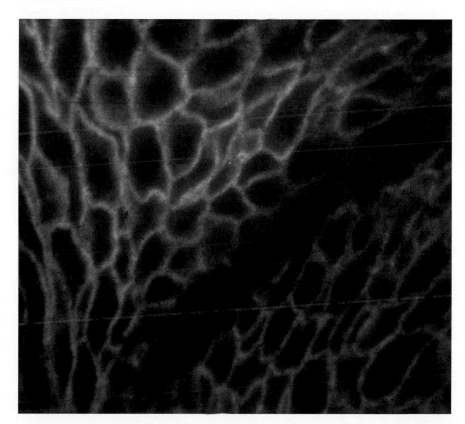

resulting in blister formation secondary to minor amounts of trauma. Diagnosis requires histopathology as well as direct and indirect immunofluorescence studies. Management includes corticosteroids, dapsone, azathioprine, mycophenolate mofetil, rituximab, and intravenous immunoglobulin. Oral lesions may be responsive to intensive topical corticosteroid therapy.

5.11.3 Linear IgA Disease

Linear IgA disease, also known as *Linear IgA bullous dermatosis*, is an autoimmune subepidermal vesiculobullous disorder characterized by deposition of IgA at the basement membrane zone. Numerous autoantibodies and target antigens have been identified. Linear IgA disease affects both children and adults; in children the course is often self-limiting while drug-related cases are more common in older adults. Oral lesions are common and clinically identical to those seen in MMP. Diagnosis requires perilesional biopsy for both histopathology and immunofluorescence studies. Management includes prednisone, dapsone, sulfapyridine, and colchicine. Intensive intraoral topical therapy as described above can be very effective.

Sources

Ayangco L, Rogers RS. Oral manifestations of erythema multiforme. Dermatol Clin 2003;21:195–205

Challacombe SJ, Setterfield J, Shirlaw P, et al. Immunodiagnosis of pemphigus and mucous membrane pemphigoid. Acta Odontol Scand 2001;59:226–34

Dagistan S, Goregen M, Miloglu O, et al. Oral pemphigus vulgaris: a case report with review of the literature. J Oral Sci 2008;50:359–62

Eguia del Valle A, Aguirre Urizar JM, Martinez Sahuquillo A. Oral manifestations caused by the linear IgA disease. Med Oral 2004;9:39–44

Escudier M, Bagan J, Scully C. Number VII Behçet's disease (Adamantiades syndrome). Oral Dis 2006;12:78–84

Grave B, McCullough M, Wiesenfeld D. Orofacial granulomatosis: a 20-year review. Oral Dis 2009;15:46–51

Hirshberg A, Amariglio N, Akrish S, et al. Traumatic ulcerative granuloma with stromal eosinophilia: a reactive lesion of the oral mucosa. Am J Clin Pathol 2006;126:522–9

Kanerva M, Moilanen K, Virolainen S, et al. Melkersson-Rosenthal syndrome. Otlaryngol Head Neck Surg 2008;138:246–51

Mignogna MD, Fortuna G, Leuci S, et al. Nikolsky's sign on the gingival mucosa: a clinical tool for oral health practitioners. J Periodontol 2008;79:2241–6

Radfar L, Wild RC, Suresh L. A comparative treatment study of topical tacrolimus and clobetasol in oral lichen planus. Oral Surg Oral Med Oral Pathol Oral Radiol Endod 2008;105:187–93

Scully C. Aphthous ulceration. N Engl J Med 2006;355:165–72

Scully C, Carrozzo M. Oral mucosal disease: Lichen planus. Br J Oral Maxillofac Surg 2008;46:15–21

Scully C, Lo Muzio L. Oral mucosal diseases: mucous membrane pemphigoid. Br J Oral Maxillofac Surg 2008;46:358–66

Scully C, Porter S. Oral mucosal disease: recurrent aphthous stomatitis. Br J Oral Maxillofac Surg 2008;46:198–206

Termino VM, Peebles RS. The spectrum and treatment of angioedema. Am J Med 2008;12:282–6

Tilakaratne WM, Freysdottir J, Fortune F. Orofacial granulomatosis: review on aetiology and pathogenesis. J Oral Pathol Med 2008;37:191–5

Woodley DT, Remington J, Chen M. Autoimmunity to type VII collagen: epidermolysis bullosa acquisita. Clin Rev Allergy Immunol 2007;33:78–84

Yancey KB, Egan CA. Pemphigoid: clinical, histological, immunopathologic, and therapeutic considerations. JAMA 2000;19:350–6

Zhu X, Zhang B. Paraneoplastic pemphigus. J Dermatol 2007;34:503–11

Chapter 6
Pigmented Lesions

Summary Unusual or abnormal coloration of the oral mucosa can arise from a variety of exogenous (extrinsic) or endogenous (intrinsic) sources. Pigmentation varies widely and may be present in a generalized fashion throughout the oral cavity or as an isolated focal lesion. This chapter discusses the etiology and presentation of pigmented lesions as well as certain systemic conditions associated with oral pigmentation. Diagnostic and treatment guidelines are provided.

Keywords Physiologic pigmentation • Exogenous pigmentation • Endogenous pigmentation • Melanin • Melanocyte • Bilirubin • Melanotic macule • Nevus • Smoker's melanosis • Addison disease • Cushing syndrome • Peutz-Jeghers syndrome • Amalgam tattoo • Hemochromatosis • Ferritin • Hemoiderin • Varix • Hemangioma • Vascular malformation • Pyogenic granuloma • Kaposi sarcoma • Hematoma • Petechiae • Osler-Weber-Rendu syndrome

6.1 Introduction

Unusual or abnormal coloration of the oral mucosa can arise from a variety of exogenous (extrinsic) or endogenous (intrinsic) sources. Extrinsic pigmentation occurs following exposure to foreign agents such as medication or heavy metals. Intrinsic pigmentation is most often secondary to an increased presence of melanin, which is produced by melanocytes in the basal layer of the epithelium. These cells are derived from neural crest tissue and migrate to the epithelium during development.

Pigmentation may be present in a generalized fashion throughout the oral cavity or as an isolated (focal) lesion. Generalized pigmentation can represent either a normal (physiologic) response (see Chap. 2) or manifestation of a pathologic process. In general, the intensity of color depends on the amount and location of melanin within the tissue. Lesions in close proximity to the surface appear brown or black, while deeper deposits appear blue. Nonmelanotic lesions may also appear pigmented. For example, bilirubin imparts a yellow color to the mucosa in patients with jaundice (see Chap. 11) and vascular lesions may appear red or blue.

6.2 Melanotic Lesions

6.2.1 Melanotic Macule

This is an isolated, flat (macular), benign, asymptomatic lesion with well-demarcated borders, and brownish-black or bluish color that is usually no larger than 1–2 mm in diameter (Figs. 6.1 and 6.2). The lower lip vermillion is affected most frequently, followed by the gingiva, buccal mucosa, and hard palate. Histologically, it is characterized by increased melanin production without an increase in the number of melanocytes (Fig. 6.3). Unless the lesion has clearly been present for a long time without change, biopsy is necessary to distinguish this from melanoma. This common lesion represents the oral counterpart to a skin freckle.

Multiple mucocutaneous melanocytic macules can be observed in the rare autosomal dominant disorder, Peutz-Jeghers syndrome. In this condition, lesions occur most commonly in the perioral region; however, freckling may also be noted on the face, extremities, and oral mucosa. This syndrome is also associated with intestinal polyps, which are generally benign but do have potential for malignant transformation. Patients are also at risk for intussusception of the bowel and should therefore be followed closely.

Diagnostic tests: None.
Biopsy: No, unless the appearance is unusual or has changed.
Treatment: None.
Follow-up: Annual examination.

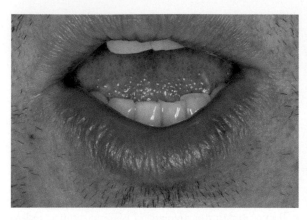

Fig. 6.1 Melanotic macule of the lower left lip. Pigmentation is light brown and the borders are well-defined.

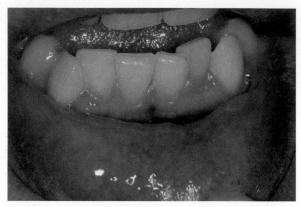

Fig. 6.2 Melanotic macule of the anterior mandibular gingiva.

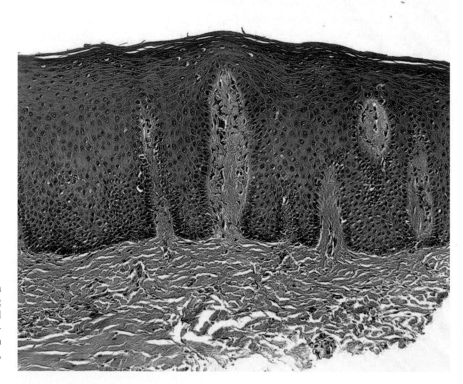

Fig. 6.3 Histopathology of a melanotic macule demonstrating a normal appearing basal cell layer with localized melanin deposition. Photomicrograph courtesy of Mark Lerman, DMD, Boston, MA.

6.2.2 Pigmented Nevus

Nevi, sometimes referred to as "moles," are seen commonly on the skin, however, can occur in the oral cavity. Pigmented nevi may appear clinically similar to melanotic macules; however, histological examination shows an increased number of melanocytes (occurring in nests or theques) in the basal epithelial layers or underlying connective tissue. They can be either flat or raised, and vary in color from brown to blue (Figs. 6.4 and 6.5). They are classified as junctional, compound, intramucosal, and blue based on the location of the melanocytes within the tissue. There is some question of malignant potential, however, this has not been clearly demonstrated. Biopsy is generally performed to rule out melanoma.

Diagnostic tests: None.
Biopsy: Yes.
Treatment: None.
Follow-up: Annual; observe for any changes in size, color, or overall appearance.

6.2.3 Mucosal Melanoma

Oral malignant melanoma is quite rare, accounting for less than 1% of all melanomas, however, it tends to be more aggressive and carries a more ominous prognosis than cutaneous melanoma. Unlike the cutaneous form where sun exposure is known to be etiologic, no risk factors have been identified for intraoral lesions. It also presents in an older age group, with an average age at diagnosis greater than 50 years. The palate and maxillary gingiva are the most common oral cavity sites; however, any questionable pigmented lesion regardless of location should be biopsied. Irregular or jagged appearing borders, change in color, rapid growth, pain, ulceration, and bleeding should arouse suspicion (Fig. 6.6). Unfortunately, most lesions are asymptomatic and may go unnoticed for a long period of time before diagnosis. Some lesions may be nonpigmented (appearing white, pink, or red), which further confounds the diagnosis.

Diagnostic tests: None.
Biopsy: Yes.
Treatment: Wide surgical excision; possible adjunctive chemotherapy.
Follow-up: Close follow-up for recurrence and metastasis.

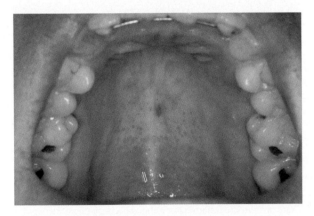

Fig. 6.4 Bluish gray nevus of the hard palate. Clinically, the lesion was slightly raised.

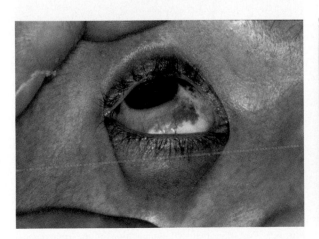

Fig. 6.5 Nevus of Ota showing striking orofacial pigmentation of the sclera. This condition is associated with increased melanin in and around the eyes.

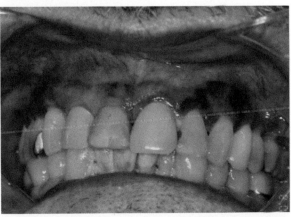

Fig. 6.6 Malignant melanoma of the left maxillary gingiva with focal, dark brown expansile area of pigmentation. Photograph courtesy of Sook-Bin Woo, DMD, MMSc, Boston, MA.

6.2.4 Inflammatory Pigmentation

Melanin is often released by melanocytes and deposited into the surrounding tissue in response to chronic irritation or inflammation. In general, this tends to occur more often in individuals with a darker baseline skin type. Smoker's melanosis is seen in heavy smokers, and is probably caused by melanocyte stimulation secondary to heat or chemical compounds in the tobacco. Lesions are typically asymptomatic and are not considered premalignant; they appear brown in color, diffuse, and flat. They occur commonly on the labial gingiva and buccal mucosa and may regress with smoking cessation (Fig. 6.7). Inflammatory pigmentation can also be seen in association with immune-mediated conditions (such as lichen planus; see Chap. 5), periodontal disease, and gingivitis (Figs. 6.8 and 6.9). Pigmentation is permanent in most cases once established.

Diagnostic tests: None.
Biopsy: No.
Treatment: None.
Follow-up: None.

6.2.5 Endocrine-Related Pigmentation

Certain endocrine conditions can result in oral pigmentation. In Addison disease (primary adrenocortical insufficiency), overproduction of adrenocorticotropic hormone from the pituitary gland causes an increase in circulating melanocyte-stimulating hormone with subsequent stimulation of melanin production. The skin takes on a bronze coloration and diffuse brown patches may be seen intraorally. Similar findings can be seen in Cushing syndrome, which involves excess production of adrenal corticosteroids. Female sex hormones may also affect pigmentation through the same pathway, with similar changes noted during and after pregnancy as well as in individuals taking oral contraceptives (Fig. 6.10).

Diagnostic tests: None; work-up for endocrine disease as clinically indicated.
Biopsy: No.
Treatment: None.
Follow-up: None.

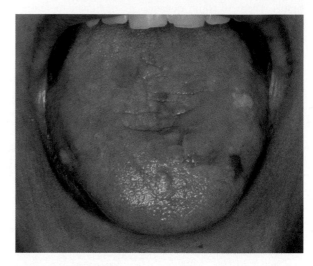

Fig. 6.8 Postinflammatory pigmentation of the tongue dorsum in a patient with chronic graft-versus-host disease (see Chap. 11). There are chronic inflammatory changes consisting of depapillation, reticulation, and erythema, as well as two focal areas of dark brown pigmentation

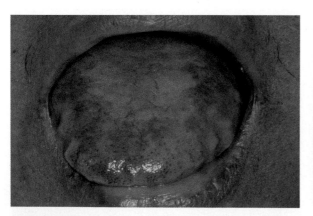

Fig. 6.7 Diffuse macular pigmentation of the tongue dorsum in an African American with a heavy smoking history.

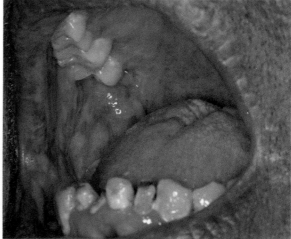

Fig. 6.9 Postinflammatory pigmentation of the right buccal mucosa in a patient with oral lichen planus.

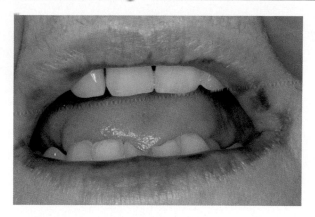

Fig. 6.10 Diffuse pigmentation of the lips in a female, most likely related to use of oral contraceptives.

6.2.6 Drug-Induced Pigmentation

This can be caused by a variety of medications, including antimalarials, antibiotics, oral contraceptives, chemotherapeutic agents, and antipsychotics (Table 6.1). The specific mechanism varies with the agent in question; it may involve an increase in melanin production or deposition of the drug or metabolite into the tissues (Fig. 6.11).

6.3 Nonmelanotic Pigmentation

6.3.1 Amalgam Tattoo

The amalgam tattoo (focal argyosis) is the most common example of extrinsic pigmentation, caused by deposition of silver-containing amalgam restoration material into the surrounding mucosa during dental extraction or placement of a filling. These are asymptomatic, blue-gray in color, and most often seen on the gingiva (Figs. 6.12 and 6.13). Diagnosis is made clinically, with biopsy reserved only for lesions that appear unusual. Biopsy shows amalgam particles within the tissue; these may also be evident radiographically. Tattooing can also be seen from graphite (pencil lead, Fig. 6.14) as well as other substances (Fig. 6.15).

Diagnostic tests: None.
Biopsy: Generally not necessary.
Treatment: None.
Follow-up: None.

Table 6.1 Medications associated with oral pigmentation

Antimalarials	Quinacrine, chloroquine, hydroxy-chloroquine, quinine
Antibiotics	Tetracycline, minocycline
Antifungals	Ketoconazole
Oral contraceptives	
Antipsychotics	Chlorpromazine (phenothiazines)
Antiarrhythmics	Quinidine, amiodarone
Chemotheraputic agents	Busulfan, bleomycin, cyclophosphamide, doxorubicin, 5-fluorouracil
Other	Zidovudine (AZT), clofazamine, carotene, chlorhexidine

6.3.2 Heavy Metals

Nonmelanotic pigmentation can be seen in cases of significant heavy metal exposure. Deposition of lead, mercury, platinum, arsenic, and bismuth occurs in a band-like distribution along the gingival margin where capillary permeability to the metals is enhanced, particularly in the presence of inflammation. These changes are not reversible with treatment of the underlying problem.

Diagnostic tests: None.
Biopsy: No.
Treatment: Treat underlying medical issue; no specific treatment for oral lesions.
Follow-up: None.

6.3.3 Hemochromatosis

This is an inherited condition of systemic iron overload characterized by increased absorption of dietary iron in the gut with deposition into body tissues. Accumulation of iron in the form of ferritin and hemosiderin eventually results in skin bronzing and organ failure including cirrhosis, diabetes, and cardiac dysfunction. Oral pigmentation can be seen in approximately 15–20% of patients, with presence of diffuse brown to gray macules.

Diagnostic tests: None.
Biopsy: No.
Treatment: None for oral lesions specifically.
Follow-up: None.

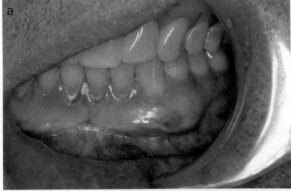

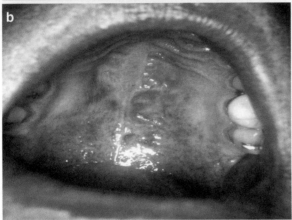

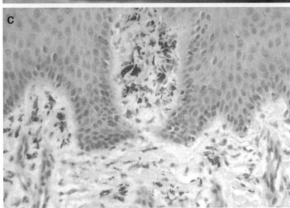

Fig. 6.11 Minocycline-induced oral pigmentation. (**a**) Focal dark gray pigmentation following gingival grafting surgery. (**b**) Diffuse brown pigmentation of the hard and soft palate. (**c**) Photomicrograph of biopsy specimen demonstrating pigment deposition in the lamina propria (Prussian blue stain). Reprinted from Treister et al. (2004), with permission from Elsevier.

6.4 Vascular Lesions

Vascular lesions appear pigmented due to hemoglobin in blood, which may be contained in underlying ves-

sels or extravasated into the surrounding tissue. Oxygenated blood in the arterial system generally appears brighter red, whereas deoxygenated blood in the venous system is more bluish-purple. The color is also affected significantly by the depth of the lesion and thickness of overlying epithelium and connective tissue.

6.4.1 Varix

Varicosities are dilated or distended veins that are seen fairly commonly in the oral cavity, most often on the ventrolateral surface of the tongue and floor of mouth. Although observed in all age groups, they are much more common in older patients. Lesions are usually superficial and painless with a classic blue to purple color and will transiently empty of blood (blanch) when manually compressed (Figs. 6.16–6.18). Occasionally small calcifications (phleboliths) form within the varix secondary to venous stasis. These may be palpable as firm nodules (Fig. 6.19) and do not need to be removed unless bothersome to the patient. Varicosities also occur on the lower lip, where excision may be indicated for cosmetic reasons or bleeding; otherwise treatment is not required.

> **Diagnostic tests:** None; clinical appearance is classic.
> **Biopsy:** No.
> **Treatment:** None unless symptomatic.
> **Follow-up: None.**

6.4.2 Hemangioma

Hemangiomas and vascular malformations are benign lesions that can be seen in the oral cavity. Hemangiomas represent a rapid proliferation of vascular endothelium arising in infancy that tends to regress (involute) with growth of the child. These are often referred to as capillary or cavernous types depending on the histological appearance. Vascular malformations exhibit a more normal appearing endothelium histologically with associated dilated or ectatic vessels. They grow proportionately with growth of the individual without involution and are classified according to the type of vessels

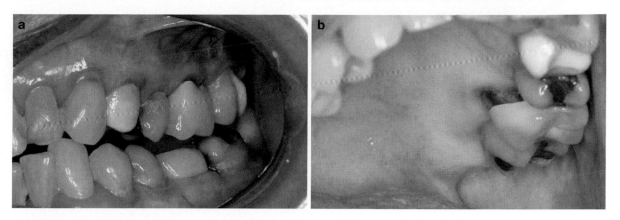

Fig. 6.12 Large amalgam tattoo of the (**a**) left buccal gingiva and alveolar mucosa, and (**b**) palate, with grayish blue diffuse pigmentation.

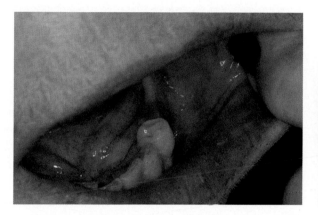

Fig. 6.13 Amalgam tattoo of the mandibular left alveolar ridge with focal gray pigmentation.

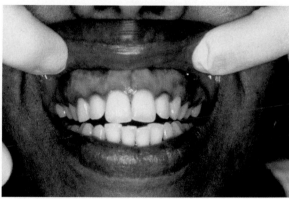

Fig. 6.15 Cosmetic ritualistic tattooing of the maxillary gingiva and alveolar mucosa in an African patient. Photograph courtesy of Sook-Bin Woo, DMD, MMSc, Boston, MA.

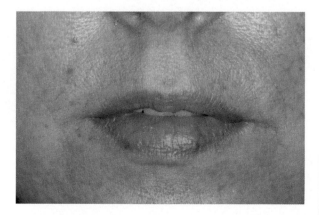

Fig. 6.14 Graphite tattoo of the right lower lip from a previous known injury with a pencil tip.

contained within the lesion (arterial, venous, capillary, and lymphatic). Clinically, both types of lesions blanch with pressure and occur most commonly on the tongue, where they can range from flat to multinodular and generally appear bluish red in color (Figs. 6.20 and 6.21). If symptomatic, they can be excised surgically or ablated using a laser.

> **Diagnostic tests:** None.
> **Biopsy:** No.
> **Treatment:** None in most cases; treatment with surgery, sclerotherapy, embolization, or laser ablation if symptomatic.
> **Follow-up:** None.

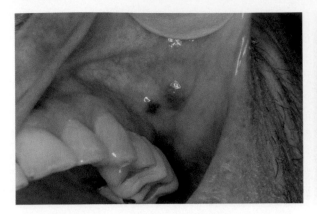

Fig. 6.16 Varix of the left maxillary vestibule.

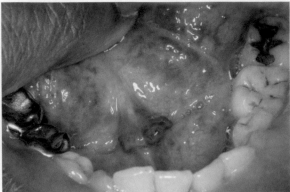

Fig. 6.19 Phlebolith formation within a varix in the area of Wharton's duct. The lesion was firm, but nontender to palpation.

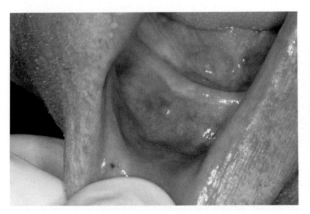

Fig. 6.17 Varix of the anterior mandibular vestibule.

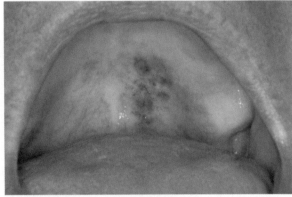

Fig. 6.20 Vascular malformation of the hard and soft palate.

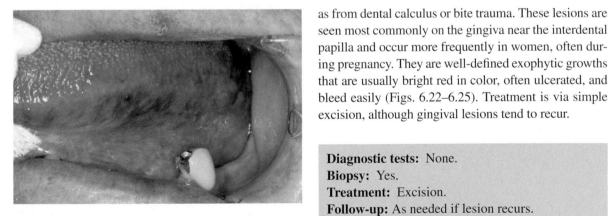

Fig. 6.18 Prominent varicosities of the ventral tongue.

6.4.3 Pyogenic Granuloma

This presents as a focal mass of benign reactive granulation tissue in response to local injury or irritation, such

as from dental calculus or bite trauma. These lesions are seen most commonly on the gingiva near the interdental papilla and occur more frequently in women, often during pregnancy. They are well-defined exophytic growths that are usually bright red in color, often ulcerated, and bleed easily (Figs. 6.22–6.25). Treatment is via simple excision, although gingival lesions tend to recur.

Diagnostic tests: None.
Biopsy: Yes.
Treatment: Excision.
Follow-up: As needed if lesion recurs.

6.4.4 Kaposi Sarcoma

Kaposi sarcoma is a vascular malignancy found almost exclusively in HIV positive individuals, however, can

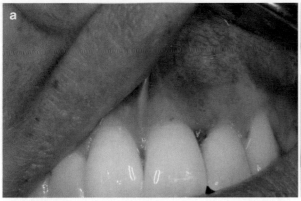
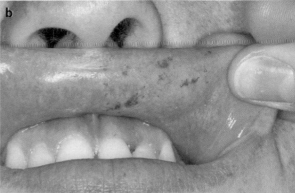

Fig. 6.21 Multifocal vascular lesions with spontaneous gingival bleeding and left sided epistaxis in a patient with hereditary hemorrhagic telangiectasia. (**a**) The lesion on the tip of the interdental papilla between the central and lateral incisors is pronounced. (**b**) Petechial lesions can also be seen in the alveolar and labial mucosa.

also be seen in other chronically immunosuppressed patients such as following organ transplantation. It has been associated with human herpes virus (HHV-8), and is seen as a marker of AIDS progression. Lesions are often multifocal and can be quite aggressive, involving the skin, lungs, gastrointestinal tract, and other organ systems. The oral cavity is frequently involved, with lesions occurring most often on the palate. The appearance ranges from flat and plaque-like to nodular with varying shades of red, blue, and purple (Fig. 6.26). They do not blanch with pressure, distinguishing them from hemangiomas. Treatment may be required for large or exopyhtic lesions if there is symptomatic bleeding or ulceration. Treatment options consist of surgical excision, local injection with sclerosing or chemotherapeutic agents, or radiotherapy. Systemic chemotherapy is reserved for severe cutaneous or disseminated disease.

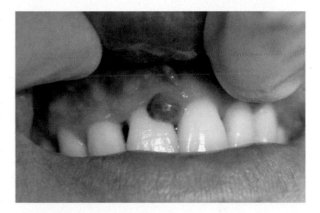

Fig. 6.22 Pyogenic granuloma of the facial gingiva with profound purplish-red color.

Diagnostic tests: Evaluation and assessment regarding underlying immune status.
Biopsy: Yes.
Treatment: Treatment of oral lesions if symptomatic.
Follow-up: Close follow-up to monitor lesions and progression of underlying disease.

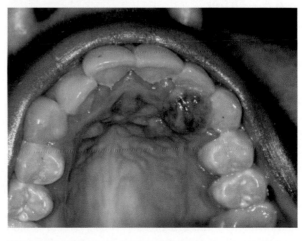

Fig. 6.23 Pyogenic granuloma of the palatal mucosa with focal ulceration.

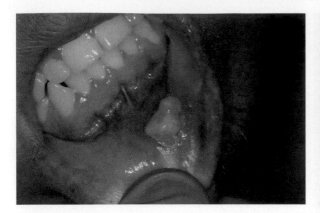

Fig. 6.24 Pyogenic granuloma of the labial mucosa. The entire surface is ulcerated.

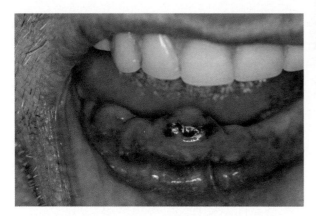

Fig. 6.25 Pyogenic granuloma of the mandibular edentulous ridge. The lesion is deeply erythematous with surface ulceration.

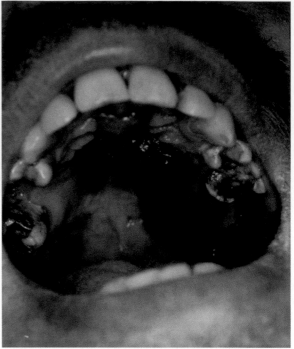

Fig. 6.26 Kaposi sarcoma of the palate in an HIV positive patient. Photograph courtesy of Sook-Bin Woo, DMD, MMSc, Boston, MA.

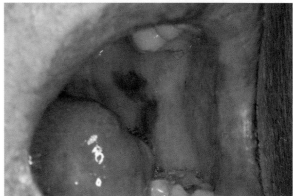

Fig. 6.27 Ecchymoses of the posterior buccal mucosa in a patient taking warfarin for anticoagulation. The lesions are clearly in the pattern of a bite injury.

6.4.5 Other

Other vascular lesions, such as hematomas, ecchymoses, and petechiae, may occur in the oral cavity as a result of minor local trauma. Lesions appear red, blue, purple, or black in color and do not blanch secondary to the presence of extravasated blood in the tissues (Figs. 6.27–6.32). They often arise in the setting of systemic blood dyscrasias but can also be seen in otherwise healthy individuals. Small dilated vessels, or telangiectasias, may be seen particularly following radiation therapy. These also occur in association with the inherited condition hereditary hemorrhagic telangiectasia (Osler-Weber-Rendu Syndrome), which is characterized by bleeding from lesions in the nasal cavity and gastrointestinal tract.

Diagnostic tests: Attempt to identify source of trauma. Laboratory testing and work-up for underlying bleeding disorder/coagulopathy as indicated.
Biopsy: No.
Treatment: None.
Follow-up: None.

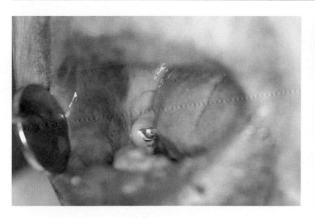

Fig. 6.28 Large ecchymosis of the right buccal mucosa in a heavily anticoagulated patient following a fall.

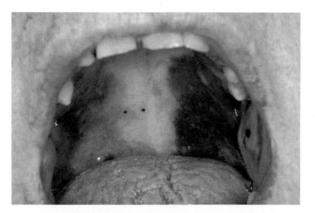

Fig. 6.29 Extensive palatal ecchymoses in a patient with profound thrombocytopenia. These lesions are asymptomatic and resulted from the mild trauma of swallowing food.

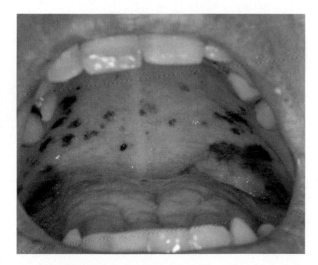

Fig. 6.30 Palatal petechiae and ecchymoses in a profoundly thrombocytopenic patient with acute leukemia.

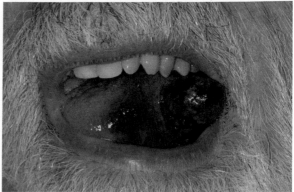

Fig. 6.31 Large hematoma of the lateral tongue in a thrombocytopenic patient with advanced multiple myeloma. The lesion was painful due to persistent trauma from chewing. With restoration of the platelet count, the lesion resolved without surgical intervention. Reprinted from Mawardi et al. (2009), with permission from Elsevier.

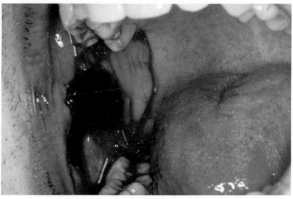

Fig. 6.32 Excessive clot formation (*liver clot*) and persistent bleeding following a 4.0-mm punch biopsy in a patient with an unreported coagulopathy. Placement of a single suture effectively closed the wound and controlled bleeding.

Sources

Dereure O. Drug induced skin pigmentation. Epidemiology, diagnosis, and treatment. Am J Clin Dermatol 2001;2:253–62

Femiano F, Lanza A, Buonaiuto C, et al. Oral malignant melanoma: a review of the literature. J Oral Pathol Med 2008;37:383–8

Giardiello FM, Trimbath JD. Peutz-Jeghers syndrome and management recommendations. Clin Gastroenterol Hepatol 2006;4:408–15

Gorsky M, Epstein JB. A case series of acquired immunodeficiency syndrome patients with initial neoplastic diagnoses of intraoral Kaposi's sarcoma. Oral Surg Oral Med Oral Pathol Oral Radiol Endod 2000;90:612–7

Jafarzadeh H, Sanatkhani M, Mohtasham N. Oral pyogenic granuloma: a review. J Oral Sci 2006;48:167–75

Lerman MA, Karimbux N, Guze KA, et al. Pigmentation of the hard palate. Oral Surg Oral Med Oral Pathol Oral Radiol Endod. 2009;107:8–12

Werner JA, Dunne A, Folz BJ, et al. Current concepts in the classification, diagnosis and treatment of hemangiomas and vascular malformations of the head and neck. Eur Arch Otorhinolaryngol 2001;258:141–9

Treister NS, Magalnick D, Woo SB. Oral mucosal pigmentation secondary to minocycline therapy: report of two cases and a review of the literature. Oral Surg Oral Med Oral Pathol Oral Radiol Endod 2004;97:718–25

Mawardi H, Cutler C, Treister N, Medical management update: Non-Hodgkin lymphoma. Oral Surg Oral Med Oral Pathol Oral Radiol Endod 2009;107:e19–e33

Chapter 7
Oral Infections

Summary Bacterial, fungal, and viral infections are frequently encountered in the oral cavity. There is no single feature characterizing infection in the mouth, and in many cases the clinical appearance may be similar to that of noninfectious conditions. Careful history taking and examination, identification of risk factors, and appropriate utilization and interpretation of diagnostic tests are critical for determining the correct diagnosis and initiating appropriate therapy. This chapter provides a rational approach to assessing, diagnosing, and managing patients with oral infections, with a special emphasis on those with underlying immunosuppression.

Keywords Caries • Cavities • Periodontal disease • Abscess • Periapical abscess • Periapical granuloma • Periapical radiolucency • Periodontal abscess • Streptococcus mutans • Ludwig angina • Necrotizing fasciitis • Mediastinitis • Trismus • Endodontic therapy • Root canal therapy • Neutropenia • Calculus • Tartar • Plaque • Periodontal disease • Furcation • Pericoronitis • Inflammatory gingival hyperplasia • Nifedipine • Phenytoin • Cyclosporine • Acute necrotizing stomatitis • Parotitis • Paramyxovirus • Mumps • Epstein-Barr virus • Cytomegalovirus • HIV • Candida albicans • Candidiasis • Thrush • Pseudomembranous candidiasis • Hyperplastic candidiasis • Erythematous candidiasis • Angular cheilitis • Aspergillosis • Cryptococcosis • Blastomycosis • Histoplasmosis • Paracoccidioidomycosis • Mucormycosis • Human papilloma virus • Enterovirus • Shingles • Postherpetic neuralgia • Ramsay Hunt syndrome • Herpes zoster oticus • Mononucleosis • Oral hairy leukoplakia • Post-transplant lymphoproliferative disease • Squamous cell carcinoma • Squamous papilloma • Verruca vulgaris • Condyloma acuminaten • Focal epithelial hyperplasia • Heck disease • Coxsackievirus • Herpangina • Hand-foot-and-mouth disease

7.1 Introduction

Bacterial, fungal, and viral infections are frequently encountered in the oral cavity. The immune system, protective components in saliva, and mucosal integrity are all key elements that work in concert to prevent the development of infection. When any of these are compromised, the resulting imbalance increases the potential for invading organisms to cause disease. Behavioral factors, including diet, nutrition, hydration, and oral hygiene, also have a significant influence on an individual's risk. Medications play an important role: immunosuppressive and immunomodulatory agents alter immune function, broad spectrum antibiotics affect the ecological balance of the oral flora, and xerogenic agents impact on the composition and flow of saliva.

There is no single feature characterizing infection in the mouth; findings range from painful swelling to mucosal ulceration to painless papules. The clinical appearance may be similar to that of noninfectious conditions. Therefore, careful history taking and examination, identification of risk factors, and appropriate utilization and interpretation of diagnostic tests (see Chap. 3) are critical. The clinical presentation of some infections may be altered in the *immunocompromised* patient: the anatomic distribution of lesions can be quite different, typical signs of infection may be

J.M. Bruch and N.S. Treister, *Clinical Oral Medicine and Pathology,*
DOI 10.1007/978-1-60327-520-0_7, © Humana Press, a part of Springer Science+Business Media, LLC 2010

diminished or absent, and standard doses of therapeutic medications may be ineffective. Failure to diagnose and initiate appropriate therapy in these patients can result in needless pain and suffering as well as progression to systemic infection.

7.2   Bacterial Infections

Oral bacterial infections are most commonly of dental origin and can progress to abscess formation with potential significant complications if left untreated. In an otherwise healthy individual, it is exceedingly rare for a nonodontogenic bacterial infection to develop within the oral cavity. Infection rarely occurs following oral surgical procedures (such as tooth extraction and soft tissue biopsy) or trauma. Infection of the salivary glands is uncommon and mucosal infection

outside of the periodontium is generally only encountered in those who are immunosuppressed.

7.2.1   Odontogenic Infections

Odontogenic infections can be broadly classified as either *endodontal,* which are characterized by infection of the dental pulp initiated by dental caries; or *periodontal,* which are characterized by infection of the tooth's supporting structures initiated by accumulation of plaque and calculus (Fig. 7.1). In both cases, the primary risk factors include inadequate oral hygiene with dental plaque accumulation. While the reasons are not entirely clear, many patients with high caries rates often have minimal periodontal disease, whereas patients with advanced periodontal disease often have few caries.

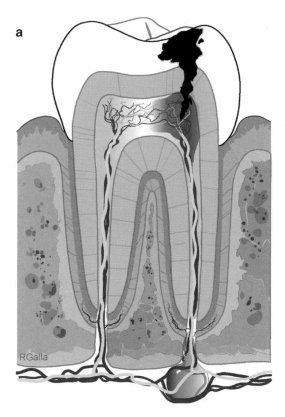
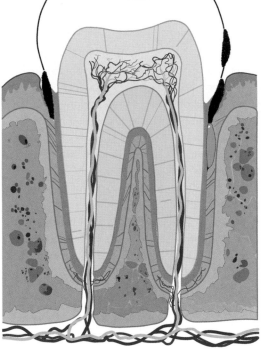

Fig. 7.1 Odontogenic infection. (**a**) Caries is seen extending through the calcified enamel and dentin of the crown with pulpal involvement. A periapical abscess has formed at a root apex (*illustrated in green*), representing extension of necrotic material from the pulp chamber into the alveolar bone through the apical foramen. (**b**) Accumulation of calculus on the crown and root surface (subgingival and supragingival; *illustrated in black*) with deepening of the gingival crevice and formation of a periodontal pocket. Note also how a periodontal abscess (*illustrated in green*) may form in this situation.

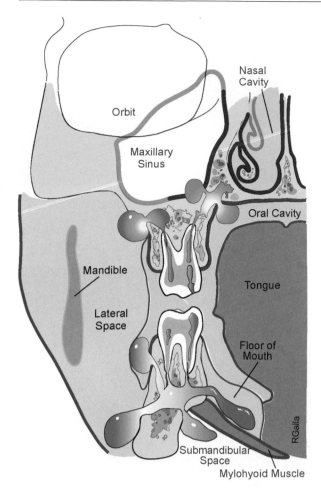

Fig. 7.2 Potential pathways of spread of odontogenic infection illustrated on a coronal diagram. Infection (*illustrated in green*) takes the path of least resistance and can emerge from the alveolar bone into the vestibule, floor of mouth, submandibular space, maxillary sinus, nasal cavity, palate, and lateral muscular space surrounding the mandibular ramus.

7.2.1.1 Dental Caries

Caries are caused by the metabolism of sugar in dental plaque by *Streptococcus mutans*, resulting in the production of acid and subsequent demineralization of the protective enamel layer. The destructive process advances inward toward the pulp with ultimate pulpal necrosis. Infected material drains from the pulp chamber through the apical foramen into surrounding bone, causing abscess formation at the root apex (*periapical abscess*). From there infection can spread to other parts of the oral cavity, face, or neck and lead to potentially life-threatening soft-tissue infections such as Ludwig angina, deep neck abscess, necrotizing fasciitis, and mediastinitis (Figs. 7.2 and 7.3). Infection in molars can result in *trismus* (limitation of mouth opening) due to inflammation of the adjacent masticatory muscles (Fig. 7.4).

Decay can form on any tooth surface, but frequently affects the occlusal surfaces of posterior teeth due to the presence of anatomic pits and fissures. The interproximal surfaces are also commonly affected because plaque can be difficult to remove from these areas. The facial surfaces near the gingival margin and exposed root surfaces are particularly susceptible because they are covered with cementum, which is much softer than enamel. Early lesions may show areas of decalcification on the enamel, and are characterized by white spots that may collapse under the pressure of a dental instrument (Fig. 7.5). More advanced lesions demonstrate obvious cavitation with brownish-black discoloration (Figs. 7.6 and 7.7). Entire sections of the tooth may fracture and exposure of the pulp chamber may be evident (Fig. 7.8).

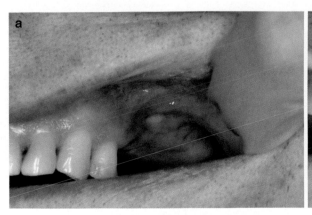
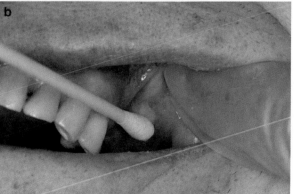

Fig. 7.3 Left buccal vestibule showing draining sinus tract from molar region; the offending tooth has been extracted. (**a**) Visible purulence; (**b**) bacterial culture obtained.

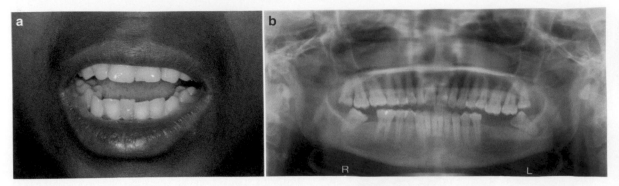

Fig. 7.4 Severe trismus in a patient with an abscessed third molar. (**a**) This is the widest opening that the patient is able to achieve. (**b**) Panoramic radiograph showing the mandibular left third molar with extensive caries and a large periapical radiolucency.

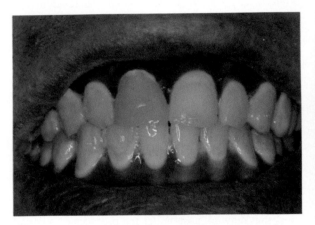

Fig. 7.5 Generalized decalcification or "white spots" along the cervical margins. Caries are most likely already present in many of these areas. The right maxillary central incisor is restored with a temporary crown made of an acrylic material.

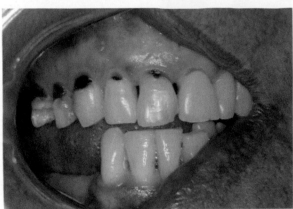

Fig. 7.7 Dark brown cervical caries. Dental caries that are longstanding or "arrested" tend to become darker in appearance over time.

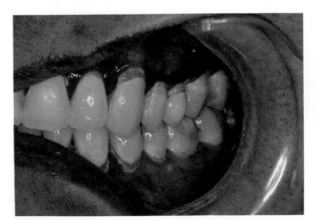

Fig. 7.6 Generalized cervical caries with clear loss of enamel and brown discoloration. This pattern of dental caries is often seen in patients with salivary gland hypofunction.

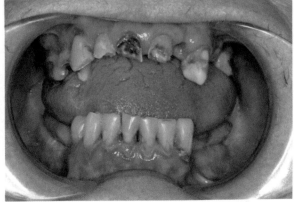

Fig. 7.8 Rampant decay in a patient several years after completion of radiation therapy for head and neck cancer. The maxillary central incisors are fractured at the cervical margin and the pulp chambers are exposed.

Intraoral radiographs are used to diagnose dental caries, which appear as distinct areas of radiolucency within the tooth structure (Fig. 7.9). These radiographs can also demonstrate the presence of a *periapical radiolucency*, indicating pulpal pathology (Fig. 7.10). Computed tomography (CT) may be indicated If extensive soft tissue swelling is present (Fig. 7.11). When dental infection is suspected, the patient should be referred to a dentist or other oral health care specialist for further evaluation.

As long as the pulp chamber has not been breached, caries can be mechanically removed and the tooth can be restored with a variety of dental materials. With pulpal involvement, endodontic therapy (*root canal therapy*) or extraction of the tooth is required. Endodontic treatment involves removal of neurovascular tissue from the pulp chamber and replacement with an inert material such as gutta-percha. In cases of localized intraoral swelling, incision and drainage may also be necessary in conjunction with definitive treatment of the tooth itself.

The only significant medical risk factor for the development of dental caries is reduced salivary function (see Chap. 8). In patients with profound neutropenia, previously latent or subclinical periapical infections can become acutely active with soft tissue swelling or localized gingival and mucosal necrosis (Fig. 7.12). Antibiotics should be given in these situations, as well as in cases of significant soft tissue swelling. Otherwise, the decision to prescribe antibiotics will depend on the individual clinical situation.

The mainstays of caries prevention involve attention to diet, maintenance of oral hygiene, and use of fluoride. Overall consumption of carbohydrate and frequency of exposure are both important. For example, an individual who ingests snacks or sugary beverages frequently throughout the day is at higher risk for caries than someone who eats only three meals per day and drinks water. Brushing with a soft toothbrush and fluoride toothpaste for 2 min at least twice daily (ideally after every meal) removes plaque accumulation and significantly reduces the risk of dental caries. Daily use of dental floss removes plaque from the interproximal regions, which are otherwise difficult areas to clean. Systemic fluoride, usually obtained through fluoridated water, is important during tooth development in children because it incorporates into the developing tooth structure and renders it less susceptible to attack from caries. Prescription topical fluoride preparations are typically reserved for individuals considered to be at high risk for caries.

> **Diagnostic tests:** Clinical exam and intraoral radiographs.
>
> **Biopsy:** No.
>
> **Treatment:** Mechanical removal of decayed tooth structure and restoration of tooth integrity. Endodontic therapy or extraction of tooth is indicated when the pulp is infected. Consider antibiotics depending on clinical presentation, in which case penicillin-group or clindamycin for 7–10 days is generally effective.
>
> **Follow-up:** Patients with dental caries should be seen by a dentist regularly following treatment of all active caries to monitor for new or recurrent lesions. High risk patients and those with rampant caries should be prescribed sodium fluoride gel 5,000 parts-per-million which can be applied by toothbrush or in soft custom-fabricated dental trays.

7.2.1.2 Periodontal Disease

Periodontal disease is caused by the accumulation of plaque and *calculus* (calcified dental plaque also referred to as *tartar*), that leads to chronic inflammation of the adjacent gingiva, periodontal attachment structures, and alveolar bone. Periodontal "pockets" form between the tooth and gingival soft tissues as

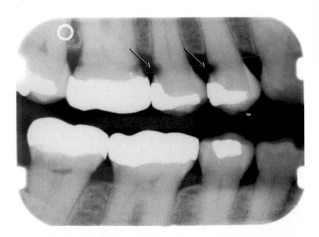

Fig. 7.9 Bitewing radiograph demonstrating interproximal decay (*arrows*) on the root surfaces of the posterior maxillary teeth. The areas of decay appear as rounded radiolucent lesions.

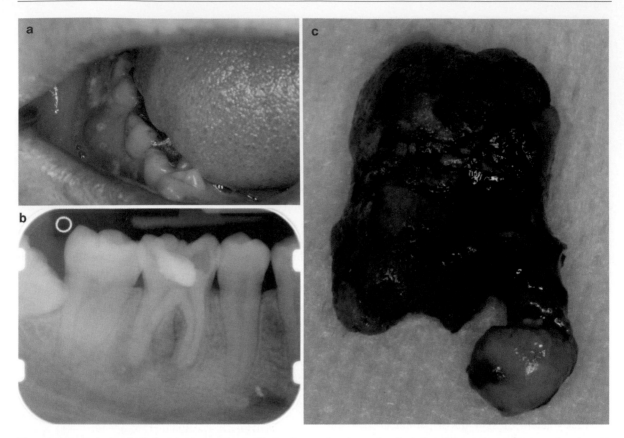

Fig. 7.10 Periapical pathology. (**a**) Abscessed mandibular first molar with adjacent gingival swelling. (**b**) Periapical radiograph (not the same patient) showing caries extending into the pulp chamber and periapical radiolucencies. (**c**) Extracted molar with attached periapical lesion; histopathological evaluation is required to differentiate between a *granuloma* versus *radicular cyst.*

the infected material migrates apically. As the pockets become deeper and more inflamed, it becomes more difficult to adequately clean these areas. Heavy smoking also contributes to inflammation of the periodontium. Signs of periodontal disease include plaque and calculus accumulation, gingival recession or bleeding, periodontal pocketing, root exposure, and tooth mobility (Figs. 7.13–7.15). Advanced periodontal disease is often associated with foul smelling breath (halitosis).

The periodontium can become acutely infected with abscess formation and swelling of the adjacent gingiva (Fig. 7.16). This is more likely to develop in areas with deep periodontal pockets and *furcation involvement* (exposure of the space between the roots of multi-rooted teeth). *Periocoronitis* is a condition in which the gingiva surrounding the crowns of partially erupted molars (usually the third molar or "wisdom tooth") becomes painfully inflamed (Fig. 7.17).

Radiographic features of periodontal disease include the presence of calculus both above (supragingival) and below (subgingival) the gingival margin, as well as loss of alveolar bone surrounding the teeth (Fig. 7.18). Generalized horizontal bone loss in all four quadrants signifies longstanding inflammation. Localized areas of vertical bony defects represent areas of advanced bone loss and are often associated with tooth mobility and an increased risk for abscess formation.

Primary management of periodontal disease includes professional *scaling* and *root planning*, with removal of calculus and inflammatory tissue from around the teeth and along root surfaces in conjunction with attention to improved oral hygiene. In more advanced cases, surgical procedures may be indicated to reduce pocket depth. Antimicrobial therapies include topical rinses, such as chlorhexidine gluconate; locally delivered antibiotics, such as minocycline injected subgingivally; and systemic antibiotics.

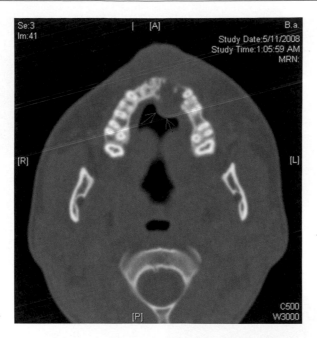

Fig. 7.11   Axial CT scan demonstrating a large abscess associated with the maxillary left lateral incisor with destruction of the palatal bone and extensive soft tissue swelling.

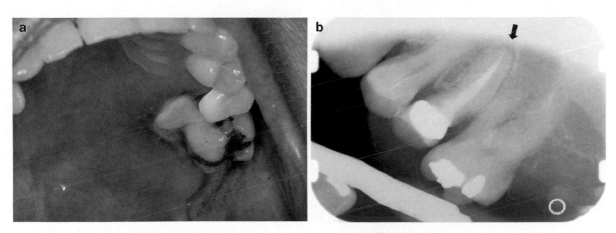

Fig. 7.12 Abscessed premolar in a patient with advanced refractory acute myelogenous leukemia. (**a**) Secondary neutropenic ulceration of the palate due to spread of infection. (**b**) Periapical radiograph showing adequate-appearing endodontic ("root canal") treatment with periapical radiolucency (*arrow*). The tooth was treated years previously and only became symptomatic in the context of profound neutropenia. (Reprinted with permission from Lerman et al. (2008); Elsevier).

Diagnostic tests: Clinical exam and intraoral radiographs.

Biopsy: No.

Treatment: Scaling and root planning and education regarding improved oral home care. In some cases antimicrobial and/or surgical therapy may be indicated. Pericoronitis should be initially managed with broad spectrum antibiotics (e.g., amoxicillin/clavulanic acid) and warm salt water rinses; extraction is necessary in recurrent cases.

Follow-up: Patients with periodontal disease typically require professional dental cleaning three to four times annually. The patient is frequently managed in conjunction with a periodontist. Home oral hygiene instruction is important. Smoking cessation should be discussed and encouraged.

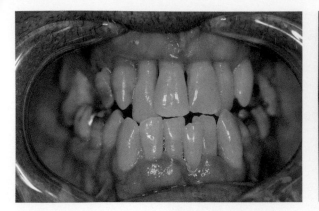

Fig. 7.13 Chronic periodontal disease. There is extensive alveolar bone loss, gingival recession, and blunting of the interdental papillae with subsequent root surface exposure.

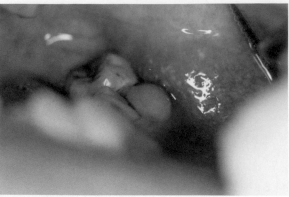

Fig. 7.16 Periodontal abscess formation with firm swelling in the buccal vestibule.

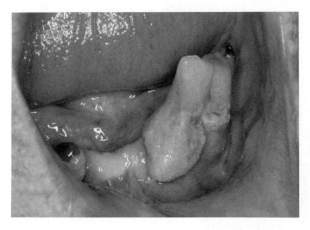

Fig. 7.14 Heavy calculus deposition on the mandibular anterior teeth. This degree of calculus formation is seen in cases of severe neglect.

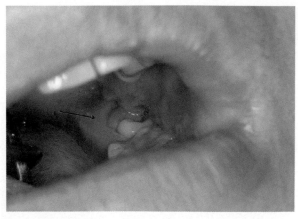

Fig. 7.17 Pericoronitis associated with the mandibular left third molar. Note inflammation and swelling (*arrow*) of the soft tissue as well as limited mouth opening.

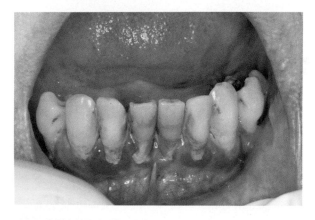

Fig. 7.15 Calculus accumulation on the mandibular anterior dentition with gingival recession and focal areas of severe inflammation.

7.2.1.3   Inflammatory Gingival Hyperplasia

Although uncommon, the gingiva can become markedly enlarged in response to localized inflammation. This can be observed secondary to periodontal disease or in response to certain medications. These include calcium channel blockers (such as nifedipine), calcineurin inhibitors (cyclosporine), and anticonvulsants (phenytoin). In all cases, poor oral hygiene is believed to be a significant contributing factor. The underlying mechanism is thought to be related to calcium regulation of collagen degradation in fibroblasts resulting in increased production of dense connective tissue. Unlike the gingival enlargement that can be seen with leukemic infiltration (see Chap. 11), these lesions are generally firm and of a normal pink color without significant associated bleeding (Figs. 7.19–7.21). Treatment includes gross debridement of plaque and calculus, which often results in partial or complete resolution. If associated with a medication, discontinuation or substitution is indicated and often effective in reducing progression of gingival enlargement. If this does not result in significant improvement, localized gingivectomy by a periodontist is indicated.

Diagnostic tests: None.

Biopsy: May be necessary for definitive diagnosis and to exclude malignancy, especially in cases where there are localized areas of prominent gingival enlargement.

Treatment: Scaling and root planning as primary therapy; patients must also maintain strict oral hygiene practices. Discontinuation of any potentially causative medication if appropriate. For lesions that do not resolve following conservative therapy, referral to a periodontist for gingivectomy is indicated.

Follow-up: None specifically indicated.

7.2.1.4 Acute Necrotizing Stomatitis

Previously referred to as "trench mouth" described in soldiers fighting on the front lines in World War I, *acute necrotizing stomatitis* is seen mainly in patients with severe malnutrition and very poor oral hygiene. It has also been observed disproportionately in patients with HIV disease. This aggressive and painful periodontal infection is caused by the convergence of very poor oral hygiene, immune suppression, and inadequate nutrition. When localized to the gingiva, the condition is called *acute necrotizing gingivitis*; if it progresses to involve the periodontium, it is referred to as *acute necrotizing periodontitis*. Rarely, this develops into a destructive and devastating infection of the hard and soft orofacial tissues resulting in a disfiguring condition termed *noma*, which is seen almost exclusively in developing countries.

Clinical features of necrotizing stomatitis include severe gingival inflammation with edema, bleeding, blunting of tissue contours, and "punched out" appearing interdental defects with varying areas of ulceration (Fig. 7.22). Necrotic alveolar bone may be evident, and heavy plaque and calculus accumulations are generally present. Intraoral radiographs demonstrate advanced bone loss with vertical defects that often

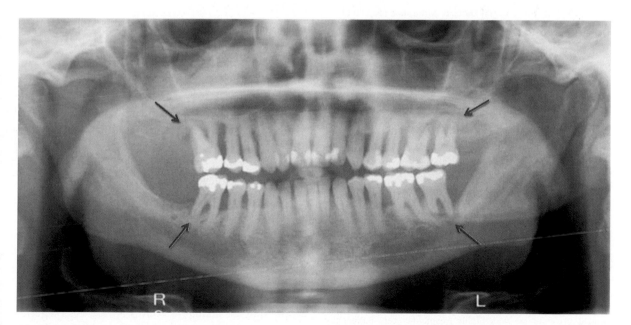

Fig. 7.18 Panoramic radiograph of a patient with advanced periodontal disease. Note advanced alveolar bone loss (*arrow*) around the posterior teeth.

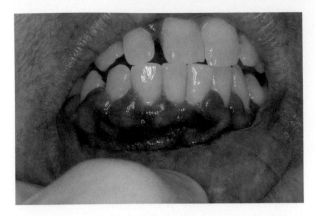

Fig. 7.19 Inflammatory gingival hyperplasia secondary to chronic periodontal disease. The changes were evident in all four quadrants and tissue was biopsied to rule out other pathology.

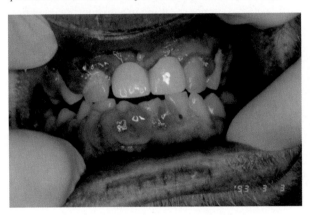

Fig. 7.20 Calcium channel blocker and calcineurin inhibitor associated gingival hyperplasia in a solid organ transplant recipient. There is considerable erythema in areas of heavy plaque accumulation. Photograph courtesy of Sook-Bin Woo, DMD, MMSc, Boston, MA

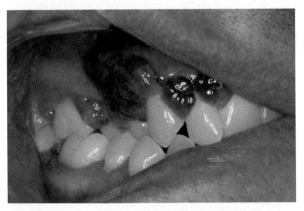

Fig. 7.21 Severe inflammatory gingival hyperplasia secondary to chronic periodontal disease with spontaneous bleeding. The clinical presentation was highly suspicious for malignancy, however, histopathological evaluation demonstrated only proliferation of benign granulation tissue.

correspond to areas of extensive soft tissue destruction. This condition is associated with a very foul odor, reflective of the extent of infection and tissue necrosis.

Treatment includes aggressive debridement and administration of antibiotics. Due to the extent and depth of infection, local anesthesia is often required for adequate removal of all plaque and calculus deposits. In addition, daily rinses with chlorhexidine gluconate provide a topical effect, and this medication is continued indefinitely after systemic antibiotics are completed. Following initial therapy, home oral care maintenance is critical to prevent recurrence. Underlying factors such as poor nutrition and immunosuppression must also be addressed.

Diagnostic tests: None.
Biopsy: No.
Treatment: Gross debridement followed by thorough scaling and root planning. A 7–10-day course of amoxicillin/clavulanic acid (250/125 mg) and metronidazole (250 mg) should be prescribed in conjunction with daily chlorhexidine gluconate rinses. Medication for pain management may be necessary.
Follow-up: Close follow-up with regularly scheduled professional dental cleanings and assessment of oral home care.

7.2.2 Parotitis

Bacterial parotitis is characterized by painful acute swelling of the parotid gland, commonly on one side. Risk factors include dehydration, salivary gland hypofunction, and sialolithiasis. In the setting of diminished salivary outflow, commensal bacteria ascend the duct in a retrograde fashion resulting in infection of the gland itself. It is usually caused by *Staphylococcus aureus*. Extraoral examination demonstrates visible fullness of the gland, often with erythema of the overlying skin and outward displacement of the ear (Fig. 7.23a). Palpation of the gland elicits discomfort, and intraoral examination may show swelling and erythema in the region of the duct orifice. Purulent discharge may be visible as well (Fig. 7.23b). Bacterial infections can also affect the submandibular glands, and are discussed in Chap. 8.

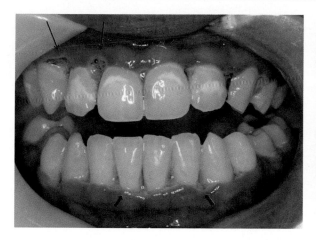

Fig. 7.22 Acute necrotizing ulcerative periodontitis in a 16 year-old female with AIDS. There is marginal ulceration of the gingiva (*short arrows*), gingival recession with loss of attachment, and crater-like interdental defects ("punched-out papillae"; *large arrows*).

Treatment includes broad spectrum systemic antibiotics, hydration to enhance salivary flow, and pain management. Drainage of the gland can be enhanced by "milking" it with gentle but steady pressure applied extraorally, which generally also improves pain. Use of sialogogues, such as sour lemon, stimulates salivary flow and helps flush out the gland. Purulent discharge should be collected for aerobic and anaerobic bacterial cultures, especially if the patient has already been treated with antibiotics without clinical improvement. Salivary stones (see Chap. 8), when present, should be removed if possible to prevent recurrence (Fig. 7.23c).

Viral salivary gland infections are characterized by nonsuppurative swelling that may or may not be painful and are usually bilateral. *Mumps* is the most common cause of viral parotitis, mediated by paramyxovirus. Given the widespread use of the MMR (measles/mumps/rubella) vaccine, this condition is encountered infrequently in most developed countries. Other viruses known to infect the salivary glands are cytomegalovirus (CMV), Epstein-Barr virus (EBV), and HIV.

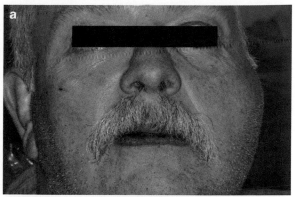

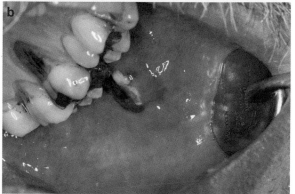

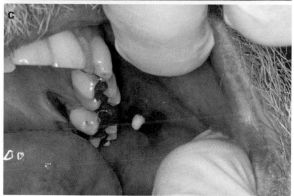

Fig. 7.23 Bacterial parotitis secondary to sialolith obstruction of Stenson's duct. (**a**) Acutely painful left-sided facial swelling. (**b**) Purulent discharge at the parotid papilla. (**c**) Delivery and removal of the sialolith. The patient felt immediate relief following stone removal.

Diagnostic tests: Culture and sensitivity of purulent discharge, especially if nonresponsive to antibiotics. CT may be ordered to evaluate for the presence of salivary calcifications or abscess.

Biopsy: No.

Treatment: Manual compression of gland to facilitate drainage of purulence via Stenson duct in conjunction with sialogogues and hydration. Broad spectrum antibiotics such as amoxicillin/clavulanic acid 875/125 twice daily for 2 weeks; up to 1 month or longer in patients with severe xerostomia. Pain medication as needed. If a sialolith is identified clinically or radiographically, consider removal of stone (see Chap. 8).

7.3 Fungal Infections

The vast majority of oral fungal infections are caused by *Candida albicans*, which is considered a component of the normal oral flora. Deep fungal infections are in comparison exceedingly rare and are generally only encountered in immunocompromised individuals; these will only be discussed briefly.

7.3.1 Oral Candidiasis

As candida species make up part of the commensal oral flora in most individuals, it is a change in the normal oral environment rather than actual exposure or "infection" per se, that results in clinical infection (*candidiasis* or *thrush*). This can be precipitated by the use of broad spectrum antibiotics, reduced salivary flow (see Chap. 8), use of topical corticosteroids (such as steroid inhalers), and immunosuppression. Oral candidiasis can be encountered in any age group; organisms colonize the mucosa resulting in a superficial infection that typically causes symptoms of soreness and burning. It is not uncommon for patients to also describe discomfort in the throat with swallowing, indicating the presence of oropharyngeal or esophageal lesions.

The most common clinical presentation is generalized patchy white to yellow spots or plaques that have a "cottage cheese" like appearance, referred to as *pseudomembranous candidiasis* (Figs. 7.24–7.26). These can be easily wiped away with gauze leaving an erythematous base with minimal bleeding. Lesions can be seen anywhere but are frequently located on the tongue, buccal mucosa, and palate. Much less

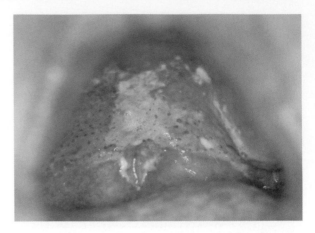

Fig. 7.25 Plaque-like pseudomembranous candidiasis of the palate in an edentulous patient whose denture hygiene was poor.

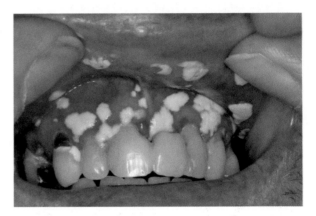

Fig. 7.26 Cottage cheese-like pseudomembranous candidiasis of the gingiva and labial mucosa.

frequently, candidiasis can present with a purely erythematous macular lesion, and is termed *erythematous candidiasis* (Fig. 7.27). Very rarely, candidiasis can present as a white plaque that does not rub away and looks clinically identical to leukoplakia (see Chap. 9); this is referred to as *hyperplastic candidiasis*. The presence of oral lesions is frequently associated with infection of the corners of the mouth, resulting in painful erythematous raw and cracked skin known as *angular cheilitis*. This is seen more frequently in edentulous patients with overclosure (collapse of jaws) and in individuals with a lip licking habit (Fig. 7.28).

Diagnosis of candidiasis can typically be made by clinical features alone. As the *hyperplastic* form cannot be distinguished clinically from leukoplakia, an incisional biopsy is required for diagnosis. Fungal culture should be reserved for lesions that are not responsive to empiric therapy. In such cases, sensitivity testing should also be requested. Clinical response to

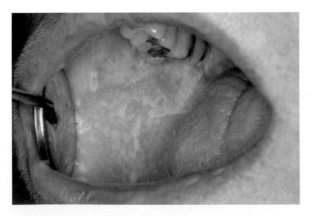

Fig. 7.24 Pseudomembranous candidiasis of the right buccal mucosa with white patches.

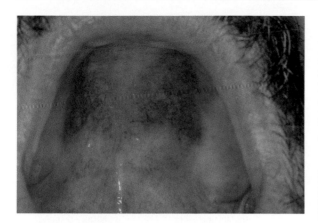

Fig. 7.27 Erythematous candidiasis of the palate.

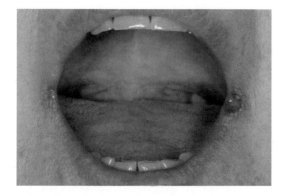

Fig. 7.28 Angular cheilitis. The commissures are ulcerated with focal erythema and cracking of the skin and vermillion.

empirical antifungal therapy, with complete resolution of signs and symptoms, confirms the diagnosis.

Primary management of oral candidiasis is with topical and systemic antifungal agents (Table 7.1). The most commonly utilized topical agents include nystatin suspension and clotrimazole troches. While both can be effective, there is greater evidence to support the use of clotrimazole troches, although some cases may not respond even with adequate dosing. Systemic therapy using fluconazole is usually highly effective. If applicable, removable dentures should also be treated, as these are frequently colonized and will continue to reinfect the underlying soft tissue (Fig. 7.25). Preparations for this are commercially available; however, a simple and inexpensive alternative is to soak the prosthesis (if it does not contain metal) overnight in a 1:10 dilution of household bleach. Angular cheilitis is effectively managed with topical nystatin/triamcinolone cream.

Management of any underlying contributing factors is important in preventing recurrence. Long-term prophylaxis should be prescribed in cases of chronic recurrent disease. Topical agents may be effective; however, systemic treatment is often easier for the patient to manage due to dosing schedules. In most cases, fluconazole given once or twice weekly is highly effective at preventing recurrent infection.

Diagnostic tests: Not generally indicated unless poorly responsive to empiric therapy, in which case fungal culture with sensitivity testing should be performed.

Biopsy: When the clinical diagnosis is uncertain, as with hyperplastic candidiasis.

Treatment: See Table 7.1. Patients with recurrent candidiasis should be treated with a prophylactic regimen.

Follow up: Close follow-up during treatment of active infection; as needed for recurrent lesions.

7.3.2 Deep Fungal Infections

Non-candidal oral fungal infections are rare and are seen almost exclusively in immunosuppressed individuals. Infections include *aspergillosis*, *cryptococcosis*, *blastomycosis*, *histoplasmosis*, *paracoccidioidomycosis*, and *mucormycosis*. Lesions typically present as deep necrotic ulcerations that can lead to localized destruction and tissue invasion as well as systemic dissemination (Fig. 7.29). Oral lesions are often accompanied by lesions within the respiratory tract, such as the lungs or sinuses, and diagnosis requires biopsy. Imaging studies should be ordered to evaluate the extent of underlying tissue involvement. Management includes aggressive systemic antifungal therapy in conjunction with surgical debridement. Despite aggressive therapy, these infections are associated with high rates of morbidity and mortality.

Diagnostic tests: Chest radiograph and advanced imaging of the head and neck (CT or MRI) to evaluate extent of involvement. Superficial cultures or swabs are of no diagnostic utility.

Biopsy: Yes; half of the specimen should be submitted in formalin and half fresh for tissue culture and advanced staining techniques.

Treatment: Antifungal therapy and surgery

Table 7.1 Management of oral fungal infections

Antifungal agent	Class	How supplied	Dispensation instructions	Regimen	Notes
Topical					
Nystatin	Polyene	100,000 U/mL suspension	One bottle (473 mL)	Swish and spit (or swallow if esophageal lesions) for 1–2 min two to three times/day. Continue until lesions resolved	Efficacy varies. If lesions do not respond, treat with systemic agent
Clotrimazole	Azole	10 mg troche	One bottle (70 or 140 troches)	Let one troche dissolve fully in the mouth, four times/day	Troches will not dissolve in patients with significant dry mouth
Nystatin/ triamcinolone acetonide	Polyene and corticosteroid	Cream	One tube (15, 30, or 60 g)	Apply a small amount to the corners of the mouth twice daily	Signs and symptoms generally respond within 2–3 days
Systemic					
Fluconazole	Azole	Tablet (100, 150, and 200 mg) oral suspension (40 mg/mL)	One month supply (30 tablets). While a full 30 day regimen is rarely required, this ensures sufficient medication in the event of recurrence or difficult to treat cases	Take one tablet once daily. A 7-day course is generally sufficient for complete clearing of candidiasis. In patients with recurrent infection (e.g., use of oral topical steroid, salivary gland hypofunction) treatment with one 100 mg tablet once or twice weekly is in most cases highly effective	True resistance to fluconazole is exceedingly rare. In the event of poor response, culture with sensitivity testing and empirically increase dose (e.g., from 100 to 200 mg). Oral suspension is useful for patients with difficulty swallowing pills. There is no evidence that topical fluconazole is any more effective than nystatin or clotrimazole

7.4 Viral Infections

A wide variety of viral infections affect the oral cavity (Table 7.2). These include members of the human herpes virus family (herpes simplex 1&2, varicella zoster virus [VZV], CMV, and EBV), human papillomaviruses, and enteroviruses. Some infections are common in normal health, while others are seen only in immunocompromised individuals. Clinical appearances are often very similar to noninfectious oral conditions and certain infections may present quite differently between the immunocompetent versus immunocompromised states. Accurate and prompt diagnosis is necessary, as the choice of appropriate management will depend on the specific organism involved, and can vary from palliative treatment alone to antiviral therapy or surgery.

7.4.1 Herpes Simplex Virus

Herpes simplex virus (HSV) is a ubiquitous virus to which the majority of humans are exposed at some point during their lifetime, usually by the teenage years but occasionally later in adulthood. The virus is transmitted through saliva by direct contact, and becomes latent in the trigeminal nerve ganglion following primary infection. Once present, the virus remains dormant and has the potential to reactivate throughout the lifetime of the individual. Subclinical viral shedding in the saliva is common even in the absence of clinically evident lesions, likely explaining to some extent the widespread prevalence of this infection in the human population. Although HSV-1 was historically considered specific to the oral cavity and HSV-2 was considered specific to the anogenital

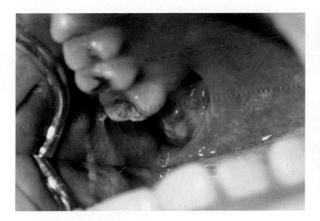

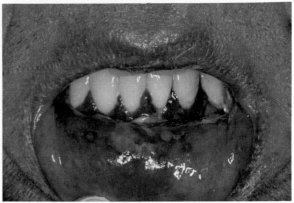

Fig. 7.29 Aspergillus infection of the maxillary sinus with invasive ulceration and necrosis of the posterior maxilla in an immunosuppressed patient following hematopoietic cell transplantation. Photograph courtesy of Mark Schubert, DDS, MSD, Seattle, WA.

Fig. 7.30 Primary herpes simplex virus infection. There are freshly collapsed vesicles, irregularly shaped shallow ulcerations, and desquamation and erythema of the gingiva.

region, either subtype can cause oral infections. This may be due to changing sexual practices as well as other factors that are not fully understood. Other than minor molecular differences between HSV-1 and HSV-2 strains, the resultant infection, natural course of disease, and treatment are exactly the same.

Primary HSV is characterized by flu-like symptoms that typically precede onset of oral lesions by 2–3 days and severe oral ulcerations that can affect both the keratinized and nonkeratinized mucosa (Fig. 7.30). The gingiva is typically very painful and fiery red in appearance. Ulcerative lesions begin as small vesicles that often develop in clusters and eventually break down to form coalescing, shallow, irregularly shaped ulcerations. The pain associated with these lesions is severe. In the absence of antiviral therapy, the clinical course of primary HSV is typically no more than 14 days with complete resolution of all signs and symptoms. There is a wide range of clinical presentations, however, and many primary infections are probably never diagnosed. A history of intimate physical contact within 1 week of developing signs and symptoms of primary HSV infection should be sought and is essentially diagnostic.

Diagnosis can often be made by history and clinical examination alone, and treatment should be initiated immediately. Viral culture or direct fluorescent antibody (DFA) testing of ulcerative lesions can confirm the diagnosis. Positive serology for HSV IgM antibodies signifies primary infection, but the presence of IgG antibodies only demonstrates prior exposure. Although

primary HSV is a self-limiting infection, early treatment with antiviral medication can reduce the severity and length of illness but will not prevent the establishment of latency. Most important is symptomatic and supportive care, as oral intake can be severely limited during primary infection due to pain. Use of systemic and topical analgesics in conjunction with hydration and nutritional support are critical aspects of management, especially in young children. Management of primary and secondary HSV infection is summarized in Table 7.2.

Once infected, the virus becomes latent in the trigeminal ganglion with the potential for reactivation or recrudescence. Well-known triggers include stress, hormonal changes, sun exposure, and trauma. Lesions are typically preceded by a prodrome, which is characterized by tingling, itching, or a painful sensation in the area where the lesion will appear. The majority of secondary lesions occur on and around the lips and nostrils and present initially with multiple small vesicles that break down and form a painful, crusted, ulceration (Fig. 7.31). Much less frequently, lesions develop intraorally, where they are limited to the keratinized mucosa. Intraoral lesions look identical to those of primary infection but are generally unilateral and limited to one specific anatomic site (e.g., tongue, gingiva, lip, and hard palate). In immunocompromised patients lesions may develop extraorally as well as intraorally, and lesions can be much more extensive; multiple areas may be affected, including both the keratinized and nonkeratinized mucosa (Fig. 7.32). Patients are highly infectious during the period of

Table 7.2 Viral infections that are known to cause oral lesions

	Type of virus	Mode of transmission	Oral lesions	Diagnosis	Management
Herpes family viruses					
Herpes simplex virus (HHV1, HHV2)	DNA	Saliva, genital secretions	Primary: • Primary herpetic gingivostomatitis Secondary: • Perioral crusted blistering lesions (cold sores) • Intraoral irregular shallow ulcers affecting the keratinized mucosa	Clinical primarily Viral culture Cytology Direct fluorescence assay (DFA) Serology	Primary: Acyclovir 200 mg five times/day for 7 days Valacyclovir 2 g once daily for 7 days Supportive care including pain control, nutritional support, and adequate hydration Secondary: Same as primary regimen, need to begin treatment at the earliest onset of prodrome symptoms Suppression: Acyclovir Valacyclovir 500 mg or 1 g once daily
Varicella Zoster virus (HHV3)	DNA	Saliva, airborne droplets	Primary: • *Varicella* or *"chicken pox,"* may present with oral ulcers Secondary: • *Herpes zoster* or *"shingles,"* unilateral intraoral ulcers identical to those caused by HSV, when cranial nerve V involved	Clinical primarily Culture Cytology DFA Biopsy	Acyclovir 800 mg five times/day for 7–10 days Valacyclovir 1,000 mg three times/day for 7–10 days Famciclovir 500 mg three times/day for 7–10 days
Epstein-Barr virus (HHV4)	DNA	Saliva	Oral hairy leukoplakia (OHL)	Biopsy	No specific treatment necessary. May respond to acyclovir or valacyclovir therapy
Cytomegalovirus (HHV5)	DNA	Bodily fluids, including saliva	Oral ulcers, typically solitary and deep, in immunocompromised patients	Biopsy	Ganciclovir 1 g three times a day until healed Valganciclovir 900 mg twice a day until healed
Human papilloma virus	DNA	Direct contact, however, lesions do not have to be present	Benign epithelial proliferations Squamous cell carcinoma of the oropharynx	Biopsy	Surgical excision If cancer diagnosed, referral to a cancer center
Enterovirus	RNA	Fecal/oral Respiratory/oral	Multiple aphthous-like ulcers, on the soft palate in particular	Clinical	Supportive care only

active lesions; however, viral shedding can occur at any time regardless of the presence of lesions.

While the diagnosis of secondary HSV infection can be made by viral culture, this is rarely necessary except for atypical cases. Treatment at the initial onset of prodromal symptoms can effectively suppress vesicle formation or reduce the severity and length of the outbreak. Topical antiviral therapy can be effective if applied frequently throughout the day, but systemic therapy is generally preferable due to better compliance.

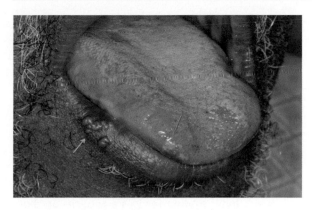

Fig. 7.31 Recrudescent herpes simplex virus infection in a patient following cardiac surgery. Note crop of intact vesicles on the lower right lip (*orange arrow*) and coalescent ulceration of the anterior right tongue (*blue arrows*).

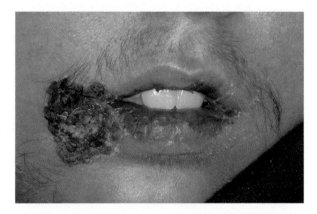

Fig. 7.32 Recrudescent herpes simplex virus infection in an immunosuppressed patient following allogeneic hematopoietic cell transplantation. The patient also had multiple ulcerations of the right lateral tongue.

Antiviral therapy is of limited utility following appearance of vesicles; lesions will heal completely within 7–10 days. For those with frequent recurrent herpes labialis, prophylactic suppressive antiviral therapy is safe and effective.

> **Diagnostic tests:** Viral culture, cytology, or DFA for definitive diagnosis. Empiric therapy should be initiated promptly when findings are clinically consistent with HSV.
> **Biopsy:** No.
> **Treatment:** Antiviral therapy and appropriate supportive care when indicated; see Table 7.2.
> **Follow-up:** As needed.

7.4.2   Varicella Zoster Virus

Primary infection with VZV results in chicken pox, following which the virus becomes latent in the spinal dorsal root ganglia. While reactivation, or *herpes zoster* ("shingles") can develop at any time, this occurs at a much higher frequency in adults greater than 60 years of age, and is thought to be related to decreased immunity to VZV. With the recent introduction of a vaccine for VZV, the epidemiology of herpes zoster infection appears to be changing; the frequency of primary infection in children is reduced; and vaccination of older adults results in a lower risk of reactivation. A rare but significant complication of herpes zoster infection is *postherpetic neuralgia* (PHN), which is characterized by burning neuropathic pain in the area of previous lesions.

Similar to recrudescent HSV infection, herpes zoster lesions are preceded by a prodrome, typically characterized by a tingling or stabbing sensation. The trigeminal nerve is involved in approximately 20% of cases and most commonly affects the ophthalmic division (V1). Lesions are characteristically unilateral and appear identical clinically to those of HSV (Fig. 7.33). The distribution of lesions follows the dermatome of the affected nerve. Diagnosis is generally made on clinical findings alone, although viral culture and DFA testing can provide confirmation. When the second or third divisions of the trigeminal nerve are affected (V2, V3), lesions may present both extraorally and intraorally. Prior to the appearance of vesicles and ulcers, intraoral herpes zoster may initially present with severe pain that can easily be confused with

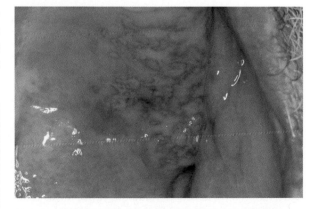

Fig. 7.33 Herpes zoster infection of the left palate. The pattern of shallow coalescing crop-like ulcerations appears to follow the anatomy of the palatine nerve branches.

odontogenic infection, sinusitis, or myofascial pain dysfunction. When cranial nerves VII and VIII are involved, facial nerve paralysis and hearing loss can occur (known as *Ramsay Hunt syndrome* or *herpes zoster oticus*). In immunocompromised patients, multiple dermatomes may be affected, lesions may present bilaterally, and disseminated zoster can develop resulting in visceral pain, organ involvement, and death.

Antiviral therapy with acyclovir, valacyclovir, or famciclovir for 7–10 days within 48–72 hours following appearance of lesions can be effective in reducing pain, promoting healing, and preventing or reducing the severity of PHN. While combined treatment of antiviral medication with high-dose corticosteroids has been evaluated to reduce the risk of developing PHN, its efficacy and clinical utility remain controversial. PHN can be managed with topical and systemic agents similar to other neuropathic pain conditions (see Chap. 10).

> **Diagnostic tests:** Viral culture, cytology, or DFA to confirm diagnosis. Serological testing is of limited utility.
> **Biopsy:** No.
> **Treatment:** Antiviral therapy with acyclovir, valacyclovir, or famciclovir at the earliest suspicion of reactivation. Topical and systemic pain management as indicated.
> **Follow-up:** PHN is rare but should be considered when pain persists in the area of lesions after resolution of lesions.

7.4.3 Cytomegalovirus

Most individuals are infected with CMV at some point during their lifetime. Initial infection is usually asymptomatic but may present as a mild flu-like illness or mononucleosis-like syndrome that is clinically identical to that caused by EBV (see below). The salivary glands become infected and provide a source of constant viral shedding. Clinically significant disease, such as pneumonia, gastroenteritis, and retinitis, due to reactivation only occurs in immunocompromised individuals. Blood tests used to evaluate CMV disease activity include antibody testing, antigen testing, shell vial assay, and qualitative and quantitative PCR.

Results from these tests may support a diagnosis, or be used as an indication to begin antiviral therapy in immunocompromised patients; however, no specific findings define infection.

Nonspecific painful oral ulcerations resembling *major aphthous* (see Chap. 5) may develop, and CMV involvement can only be diagnosed by biopsy (Fig. 7.34). Histopathology demonstrates enlarged cells within the vascular endothelial cells in the connective tissue with intranuclear inclusions that have a classic "owl's eye" appearance; immuohistochemistry and in situ hybridization for CMV antigens are both useful tests for confirmation of the diagnosis. Treatment with ganciclovir and valganciclovir are both highly effective in managing CMV disease.

> **Diagnostic tests:** Quantitative CMV viral load testing may help support a diagnosis of CMV-induced oral ulcerations. The relationship is unclear and results must be interpreted carefully. Surface cultures, as are used for the diagnosis of HSV, are ineffective given the location of CMV deep in the connective tissue.
> **Biopsy:** Yes. A sample should also be submitted fresh in viral culture medium.
> **Treatment:** Ganciclovir or valganciclovir. Blood tests to rule out secondary pancytopenia.
> **Follow-up:** Patients should be followed carefully to assess for healing of oral lesions.

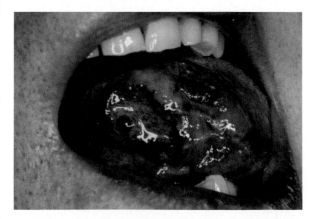

Fig. 7.34 Cytomegalovirus infection of the tongue in an HIV positive patient with multiple large, penetrating ulcers. Incisional biopsy demonstrated cytopathological changes and immunohistochemistry confirmed presence of the virus. Photograph courtesy of Sook-Bin Woo, DMD, MMSc, Boston, MA.

7.4.4 Epstein-Barr Virus

Similar to CMV, most humans are exposed to EBV. Primary infection (*acute infectious mononucleosis*) is most commonly seen in adolescents and young adults; when symptomatic it is characterized by sore throat, fever, and lymphadenopathy. Diagnosis includes (a) lymphocytosis, (b) atypical lymphocytes on peripheral smear, and (c) positive EBV serology. The salivary glands and oropharyngeal lymphoid tissues become infected and are responsible for constant shedding in saliva during latency, which is most commonly responsible for viral transmission.

B lymphocytes are also an important site of infection and latency. EBV is associated with endemic Burkitt lymphoma, nasopharyngeal carcinoma, and non-Hodgkin lymphoma, including posttransplant lymphoproliferative disease. The only oral condition that is specifically attributed to EBV is *oral hairy leukoplakia* (OHL), a benign condition characterized by painless white plaques on the ventrolateral tongue (see Chaps. 4 and 11). OHL is only seen in immunosuppressed individuals and has primarily been reported in association with HIV disease. Biopsy shows classic EBV-associated viral cytopathic changes in the superficial epithelium characterized by nuclear clearing and peripheral margination of chromatin (nuclear beading) caused by EBV viral replication. In situ hybridization can further confirm the presence of EBV in the tissue. Once diagnosed, treatment is not necessary; however, antiviral therapy with acyclovir can be effective for clinical resolution of lesions. This should not be confused with *leukoplakia*, which is not EBV associated and is considered premalignant (see Chap. 9).

> **Diagnostic tests:** EBV serology and CBC for diagnosis of primary infectious mononucleosis. HIV testing indicated if OHL suspected.
> **Biopsy:** Yes, for OHL.
> **Treatment:** Acyclovir can be effective for OHL.
> **Follow-up:** None specific for OHL; the patient's underlying medical condition should be followed carefully.

7.4.5 Human Papilloma Virus

Human papilloma virus (HPV) is a ubiquitous virus with over 100 identified subtypes. It is associated with both benign and malignant epithelial growths of the aerodigestive and anogenital mucosa. Transmission is by direct contact and prevalence in the population is estimated to be at least 50%. The most common subtypes associated with benign mucosal proliferative lesions are 2, 4, 6, 11, 13, and 32. Subtypes 16 and 18 have been associated with oropharyngeal *squamous cell carcinoma* as well as cancer of the cervix (see Chap. 9). While an HPV vaccine is now available for women for the prevention of cervical cancer, it has not been evaluated with respect to oropharyngeal carcinoma and is not FDA approved for use in males. The association of various sexual behaviors with primary infection, mechanisms of latency, and risk factors for the development of oral lesions are largely unknown.

Oral lesions caused by HPV infection include *squamous papilloma*, *verruca vulgaris*, *condyloma acuminaten*, and *focal epithelial hyperplasia* (or *Heck disease*; Figs. 7.35–7.38). While differences exist clinically between these lesions, they are all characterized by well-defined epithelial proliferations that are pink to white in color, ranging from 1.0 mm to 1.0 cm in diameter, often with a pebbly or "wart-like" surface. Lesions, although painless, may be subject to trauma from the dentition, can be annoying, and may have

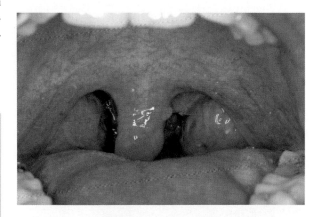

Fig. 7.35 Squamous papilloma (*arrow*) on the lateral aspect of the uvula. The lesion is well-defined with a characteristic "papillary" or pebbly texture and normal pink color.

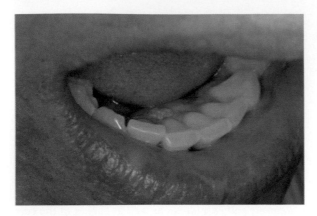

Fig. 7.36 Verruca vulgaris of the anterior lingual gingiva. The lesion is whiter than the surrounding tissue, with prominent hair-like projections.

social consequences when located on the lips or tongue. In immunocompromised patients, in particular those with HIV infection, multiple lesions often occur resulting in a condition called *papillomatosis* (Fig. 7.39). None of these lesions are considered to have any malignant potential.

Diagnosis is primarily based on clinical appearance; however, lesions may need to be biopsied to rule out dysplasia or malignancy, especially in patients who are at increased risk for oral cancer. Lesions are characterized histopathologically by marked epithelial hyperplasia and koilocytosis. Management of solitary lesions is by simple surgical excision. Treatment of multiple lesions can be more challenging and approaches include surgery, cryotherapy, laser ablation, and intralesional interferon-alpha therapy; unfortunately recurrence is common in these cases. Lesions on the lip and vermillion border (but not intraoral mucosa) may be treated with topical immunomodulatory (imiquimod) or antineoplastic (5-fluorouracil) agents, although results are variable.

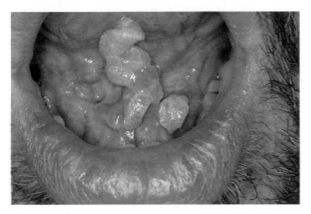

Fig. 7.37 Large condyloma acuminaten of the ventral tongue.

Diagnostic tests: None.
Biopsy: Yes, to rule out malignancy. HPV typing is not typically performed as this is of limited clinical utility with oral lesions.
Treatment: Surgical excision.
Follow-up: As needed.

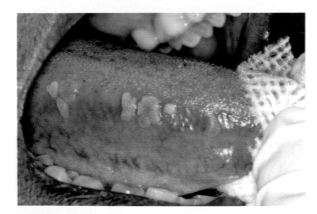

Fig. 7.38 Focal epithelial hyperplasia with multiple flat pink papillary lesions on the lateral tongue. Photograph courtesy of Sook-Bin Woo, DMD, MMSc, Boston, MA

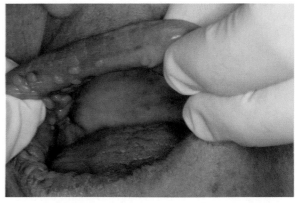

Fig. 7.39 Papillomatosis with numerous clustered squamous papillomas of the anterior oral cavity in an HIV positive patient.

7.4.6 Enterovirus

Enteroviruses belong to the Picornaviridae (small RNA virus) family of viruses and include, among many others, coxsackievirus. *Herpangina* and *hand-foot-and-mouth disease* are mediated by coxsackievirus and are both characterized by painful oropharyngeal ulcers (Fig. 7.40). Enteroviruses are transmitted primarily by the fecal–oral route, but may be transmitted by aerosolized saliva droplets as well during the acute phase of infection. Outbreaks tend to occur during the summer and fall, but in temperate climates can occur year round. Regular hand washing is the most effective preventive measure. The incubation period is 3–7 days, followed by acute onset of variable flu-like symptoms (sore throat, dysphagia, fever, and malaise), although in many cases infection is entirely subclinical. While more common in children, enterovirus infection can present at any time during life.

Herpangina is characterized by multiple small vesicles on the soft palate and tonsillar pillars that rapidly break down to form aphthous-like ulcers. Oral lesions may be more widespread in *hand-foot-and-mouth disease* and are accompanied by cutaneous vesicles. The infection is self-limiting, with systemic symptoms typically resolving within several days and oral lesions healing within 7–10 days. In most cases diagnosis is made by clinical findings alone, although various tests are available for atypical cases or for epidemiological purposes (e.g., culture, serology, and PCR). There is no specific antiviral therapy for enterovirus infection; supportive care including pain management, hydration, and soft diet should be provided until lesions and symptoms resolve.

> **Diagnostic tests:** None; diagnosis is made based on characteristic clinical features.
> **Biopsy:** No.
> **Treatment:** Supportive care measures.
> **Follow-up:** None.

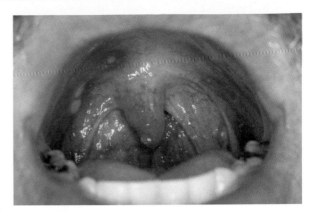

Fig. 7.40 Coxsackie virus infection with multiple shallow minor aphthous-like ulcers of the posterior soft palate and uvula with associated erythema.

Sources

Arduino PG, Porter SR. Herpes simplex virus type 1 infection: overview on relevant clinico-pathological features. J Oral Pathol Med 2008;37:107–21

Enwonwu CO, Falkler WA, Idigbe EO. Oro-facial gangrene (noma/cancrum oris): pathogenetic mechanisms. Crit Rev Oral Biol Med 2000;11:159–71

Gnann JW, Whitley RJ. Herpes zoster. N Engl J Med 2002;347:340–6

Horning GM. Necrotizing gingivostomatitis: NUG to noma. Compend Contin Educ Dent 1996;17:951–4

Hosseini SM, Borghei P. Rhinocerebral mucormycosis: pathways of spread. Eur Arch Otorhinolaryngol 2005;262: 932–8

Lerman M, Laudenbach J, Marty F, et al. Management of oral infections in cancer patients. Dental Clinics of North America 2008; 52:129–53

Nahlieli O, Bar T, Shacham R, et al. Management of chronic recurrent parotitis: current therapy. J Oral Maxillofac Surg 2004;62:1,150–5

Sitheeque MA, Samaranayake LP. Chronic hyperplastic candidosis/candidiasis (candidal leukoplakia). Crit Rev Oral Biol Med 2003;14:253–67

Sweeney CJ, Gilden DH. Ramsay Hunt syndrome. J Neurol Neurosurg Psychiatry 2001;71:149–54

Woo SB, Challacombe SJ. Management of recurrent oral herpes simplex infections. Oral Surg Oral Med Oral Pathol Oral Radiol Endod 2007;103:S12e1–8

Chapter 8
Salivary Gland Disease

Summary Saliva serves a variety of important functions, many of which are not appreciated until salivary flow decreases. A wide spectrum of pathologic conditions, including inflammatory, infectious, and neoplastic, affect the major and minor salivary glands, resulting in potentially significant morbidity and diminished quality of life for the patient. This chapter provides a review of conditions affecting the salivary glands, with attention to the more common entities that are likely to be encountered in clinical practice along with relevant practical treatment guidelines.

Keywords Saliva • Mucocele • Ranula • Mylohyoid muscle • Mucus retention cyst • Sialadenitis • Sialolithiasis • Sialagogue • Necrotizing sialometaplasia • Sialosis • Xerostomia • Sjögren syndrome • Sicca syndrome • Lymphoma • Radiation therapy • Osteoradionecrosis • Radioactive iodine • Neoplasia • Pleomorphic adenoma • Warthin tumor • Mucoepidermoid carcinoma • Adenoid cystic carcinoma • Acinic cell carcinoma • Polymorphous low-grade carcinoma

8.1 Introduction

Saliva serves a variety of important functions, many of which are not appreciated until salivary flow decreases. Lubrication of tissue surfaces and presence of salivary digestive enzymes, such as amylase and lipase, help initiate and facilitate mastication, deglutition, and digestion. Surface lubrication is also important in protecting the mucosa from mechanical trauma and enhancing taste receptor function. Salivary buffers, enzymes, and antibodies provide protection against microorganisms, caries, and demineralization of tooth enamel.

A variety of pathologic conditions, including inflammatory, infectious, and neoplastic, affect the major and minor salivary glands, resulting in potentially significant morbidity and diminished quality of life for the patient. An understanding of the anatomy and physiology is helpful in being able to accurately recognize and treat these conditions.

8.2 Mucus Extravasation and Retention Phenomena

8.2.1 Mucocele

Rupture of a minor salivary gland duct, most commonly on the inner aspect of the lower lip, may cause extravasation of mucin into the surrounding tissues (Fig. 8.1). There is usually no obvious inciting event although the patient may recall an episode of minor trauma (such as biting the lip) prior to its appearance. These lesions are typically painless, dome-shaped, and fluctuant; they appear blue in color secondary to the presence of mucin under the mucosa (Fig. 8.2). They are subject to repetitive local trauma once formed, particularly if large or bulky, and may increase in size during mealtimes. Occurrence on the palate is unusual; lesions in this area present as smaller, clear colored vesicular swellings that may rupture and be painful (Fig. 8.3). Mucoceles sometimes resolve spontaneously, however, usually require surgical excision.

J.M. Bruch and N.S. Treister, *Clinical Oral Medicine and Pathology*,
DOI 10.1007/978-1-60327-520-0_8, © Humana Press, a part of Springer Science+Business Media, LLC 2010

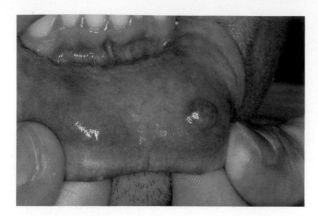

Fig. 8.1 Mucocele of the lower lip. The lesion is dome-shaped with a slightly blue hue and entirely normal surrounding mucosa.

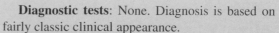

Diagnostic tests: None. Diagnosis is based on fairly classic clinical appearance.

Biopsy: Not needed unless diagnosis is uncertain.

Treatment: Excision if lesion persists or is bothersome.

Follow-up: None.

8.2.2 Ranula

This is a specific type of mucocele that arises in the anterolateral floor of mouth and represents extrusion of mucus from the sublingual gland. These are generally larger than mucoceles occurring in other locations; the tongue on the affected side may become elevated, making speaking and eating difficult (Fig. 8.4). The appearance has been likened to that of a frog's belly, hence the derivation of the name from the Latin term for frog (*rana*). They can become quite large and "plunge" below the mylohyoid muscle into the upper neck with subsequent visible neck swelling. Treatment is generally surgical and often includes removal of the feeding sublingual gland to prevent recurrence. Simple marsu-pialization, or "un-roofing," of the lesion often results in unacceptable rates of recurrence.

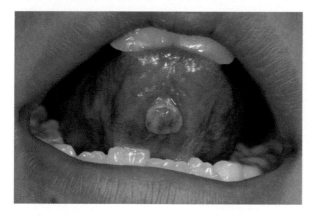

Fig. 8.2 Mucocele of the anterior ventral tongue. The lesion appears white due to ulceration from chronic trauma.

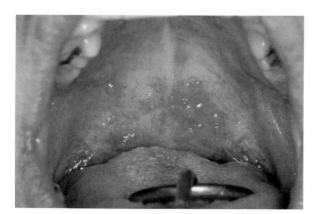

Fig. 8.3 Multiple superficial mucoceles of the palate in a patient with chronic graft-versus-host disease. Mucoceles of the palate are rare and quickly rupture.

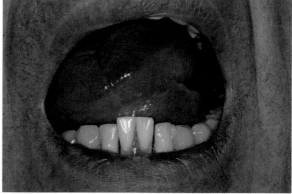

Fig. 8.4 Ranula of the left floor of mouth with notable elevation of the tongue. Note that the patient has a removable partial denture replacing the two mandibular central incisors.

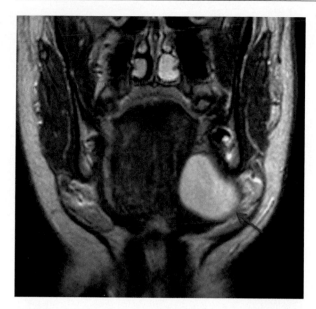

Fig. 8.5 MRI of a ranula demonstrating the extent of the lesion and displacement of the tongue. The mylohyoid muscle is not breached.

> **Diagnostic tests**: Usually none, as the clinical diagnosis is generally sufficient; imaging studies (CT, MRI; Fig. 8.5) can be obtained in cases of plunging ranula.
> **Biopsy**: No.
> **Treatment**: Surgical excision. Removal of the feeding salivary gland is also recommended (usually the sublingual, however, submandibular and minor salivary glands can be involved).
> **Follow-up**: Routine post-surgical evaluation.

8.2.3 Mucus Retention Cyst

Also called salivary duct cysts, mucus retention cysts are distinguished from mucoceles by the histologic presence of a true epithelial lining. These lesions are much less common than mucoceles although they often appear clinically similar and are usually painless. They can occur in any of the major or minor salivary glands and probably result from ductal obstruction and dilatation rather than trauma. Intraorally, they are seen most commonly in the floor of mouth, buccal mucosa, and upper lip. Treatment is surgical and recurrence is unlikely.

> **Diagnostic tests**: None.
> **Biopsy**: No.
> **Treatment**: Surgical excision.
> **Follow-up**: None.

8.3 Sialadenitis

Inflammatory conditions of the salivary glands generally present with pain and swelling of the affected gland, and are most often caused by ductal obstruction with secondary bacterial infection due to decreased salivary flow and stasis of secretions. Infection of the salivary glands is also discussed in Chap. 7.

8.3.1 Sialolithiasis

Calculi, or "stones," can develop within the salivary ducts from calcium salts that precipitate out of saliva in concentric layers around an initial nidus of debris. They occur most commonly in the submandibular gland, possibly due to the higher viscosity of the saliva in combination with a relatively long and tortuous course of the duct. The patient typically complains of episodic painful swelling in the region of the gland, which can be quite severe and tends to be more pronounced with food intake. A stone may be palpated on exam or visualized radiographically (Fig. 8.6); most salivary gland stones are radioopaque. On exam, the gland should be gently compressed, or "milked," to assess for adequacy of salivary flow from the gland as well as presence of purulence in the saliva.

Treatment involves massage of the gland, hydration, and use of sialagogues (such as sour lemon drops) to promote forward movement of secretions. Antibiotics may also be necessary to treat secondary infection. Small stones may pass on their own or be removed intraorally from the duct orifice. Increasing success has been reported using minimally invasive endoscopic techniques for this. Some institutions have reported use of shock wave lithotripsy; however, this is not widely available. Large stones may require removal of the gland itself via an extraoral approach.

Diagnostic tests: Only as clinically indicated. Plain radiographs of the anterior floor of mouth may be obtained to evaluate the number and size of stones within the duct; CT is useful to evaluate larger stones in the gland parenchyma or hilum (area where main duct joins body of gland), or to rule out abscess or tumor if suspected. Sialography is no longer commonly used, however, may be indicated in situations where a detailed image of internal ductal anatomy is desired.

Biopsy: No.

Treatment: Sialagogues, manual massage of gland, maintain hydration, analgesics, and antibiotics if infection is present. Intraoral removal of stone if it does not pass spontaneously and is accessible; surgical removal of gland if necessary.

Follow-up: As needed.

8.3.2 Necrotizing Sialometaplasia

This is a rare inflammatory condition of unclear etiology that affects the palatal minor salivary glands. It may possibly result from local ischemia and necrosis of these glands with subsequent painful swelling and ulceration that often appears clinically suspicious for malignancy (Fig. 8.7). Lesions are generally present on the posterolateral hard palate, however, can arise at any site where minor salivary tissue is found. Biopsy is indicated to establish the diagnosis, although even the histopathologic appearance can be mistaken for carcinoma. Once the benign nature of the lesion has been established, no further treatment is required, as it will heal on its own over a period of many weeks.

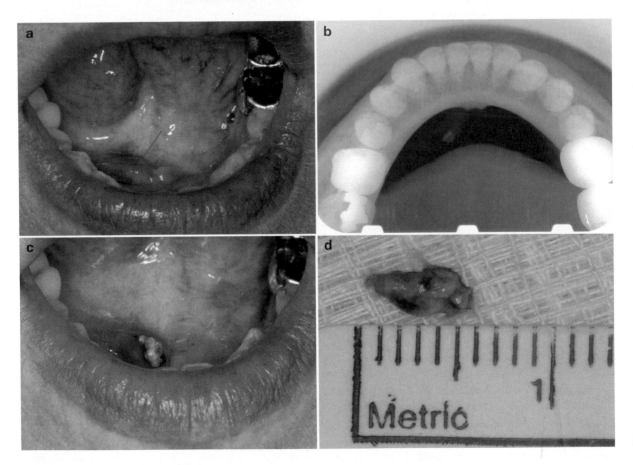

Fig. 8.6 Sialolith formation near the orifice of Wharton's duct. (**a**) Swelling and erythema of the right sublingual papilla. (**b**) Mandibular occlusal film showing a well-defined radiopacity. (**c**) Delivery of the stone following a small lengthwise incision. (**d**) Gross pathology of the sialolith following removal.

Diagnostic tests: None.
Biopsy: Biopsy to rule out malignancy.
Treatment: None.
Follow-up: None.

8.4 Sialadenosis (sialosis)

Noninflammatory enlargement of the major salivary glands, primarily the parotid, can be seen in association with a variety of systemic disorders including alcoholism, diabetes, malnutrition, and bulimia. This is generally bilateral and painless, and evolves slowly over time. Histologically, acinar hypertrophy is seen along with possible fatty infiltration. The etiology is unknown, however, may be related to inappropriate autonomic nervous system stimulation.

Diagnostic tests: Evaluate for an underlying systemic disorder, including endocrinopathy, nutritional deficiencies, alcoholism, and eating disorder. Consider imaging to rule out tumor if suspected, especially if unilateral.
Biopsy: No.
Treatment: Treatment of underlying condition.
Follow-up: As needed.

8.5 Xerostomia

Xerostomia is defined as the subjective complaint of oral dryness, which can be due to either true salivary gland hypofunction or a perception of dryness despite apparently normal salivary flow. Quantitative measurement of salivary flow is not routinely performed, therefore the diagnosis relies on visualization of salivary flow from duct orifices, pooling of saliva in the floor of mouth, and subjective assessment of mucosal moistness. Common symptoms of true salivary gland hypofunction consist of difficulty chewing or swallowing, altered taste, pain or burning sensation, and increased viscosity of the saliva. Patients may have problems wearing their dentures. Findings on exam include erythema and tenderness of the mucosa, fissuring and atrophy of the tongue dorsum, candidiasis, and potentially aggressive dental decay. Patients with complaint of xerostomia and objectively normal salivary function describe a sensation of dryness but do not typically exhibit associated physical findings. Specific causes of xerostomia are discussed further below. Treatment is symptomatic, with use of various topical products aimed at increasing mucosal lubrication and moistness. Patients should maintain adequate hydration. They may also find use of salivary stimulants such as sugar-free candy or gum to be useful. Systemic medications, primarily consisting of cholinergic agonists, are also available to enhance production of saliva; however, these may produce adverse side effects. Fluoride treatments should be given regularly to limit caries.

Diagnostic tests: The diagnosis is based on clinical exam. Sialometry is used rarely, and mainly for research purposes.
Biopsy: No.
Treatment: Hydration, OTC mucosal lubricants/saliva substitutes, and sialagogues (sugar-free candy/gum). Daily fluoride treatments. Medications: pilocarpine and cevimeline.
Follow-up: As needed.

8.5.1 Sjögren Syndrome

This is a systemic autoimmune condition affecting salivary and lacrimal gland tissue that is seen primarily in middle-aged women. Clinical manifestations of dry eyes and mouth are referred to as *sicca syndrome*, which may occur in conjunction with other autoimmune diseases such as rheumatoid arthritis and lupus (Fig. 8.8). Diffuse nontender enlargement of the major salivary glands may be present (Fig. 8.9). Histologically, focal lymphocytic

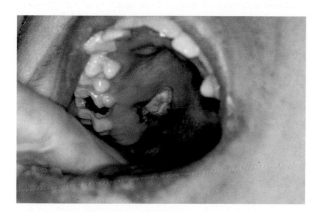

Fig. 8.7 Necrotizing sialometaplasia of the hard palate with erythema, ulceration, and focal soft tissue necrosis. Photograph courtesy of Sook-Bin Woo, DMD, MMSc, Boston, MA

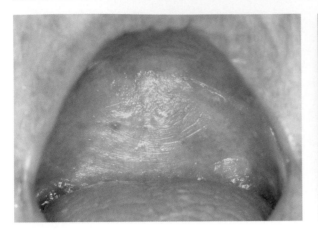

Fig. 8.8 Desiccated and atrophic palatal mucosa in a patient with xerostomia secondary to Sjögren syndrome.

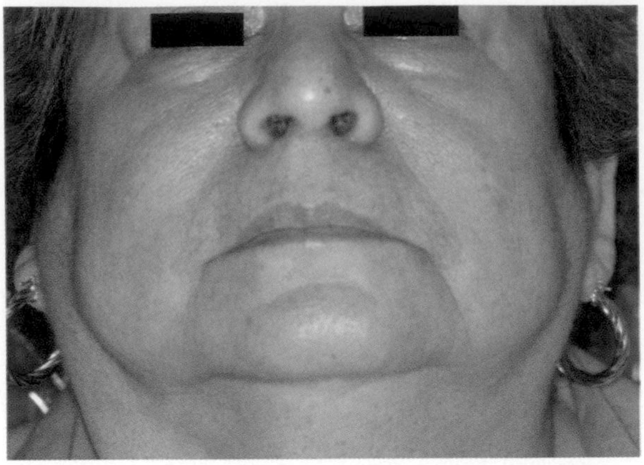

Fig. 8.9 Parotid enlargement in a patient with advanced Sjögren syndrome. Such patients should be evaluated for lymphoma.

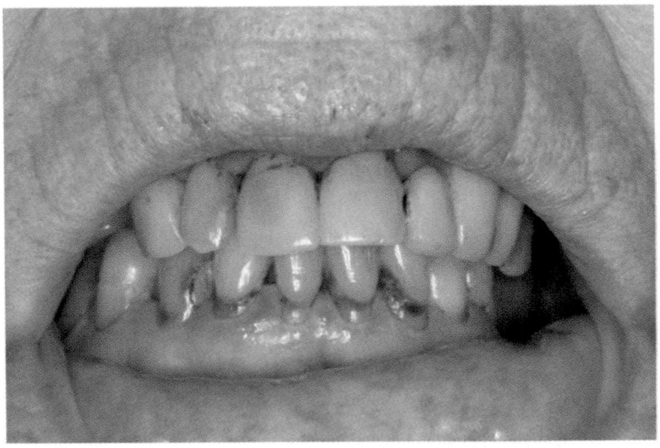

infiltration of salivary gland tissue is seen with atrophy of acini and fibrosis. Biopsy of lower lip minor salivary glands or the parotid gland is used to confirm the diagnosis along with measurement of antinuclear antibodies (ANA), SS-A (anti-Ro), and SS-B (anti-La); these tests are often, but not always, positive in Sjögren syndrome. Patients are at increased risk for lymphoma, and should be monitored for this. Treatment is nonspecific and supportive, with use of saliva substitutes, sialagogues, and fluoride treatments to minimize caries (Fig. 8.10).

> **Diagnostic tests**: Measurement of inflammatory and immune markers: ESR, ANA, RF, SS-A, and SS-B. Opthalmologic evaluation and measurement of lacrimal flow (Schirmer test).
> **Biopsy**: Biopsy of lower lip minor salivary glands or parotid.
> **Treatment**: Symptomatic and supportive as discussed above under "xerostomia"; opthalmological management of eye symptoms with artificial tears and medicated eyedrops.
> **Follow-up**: Regular follow-up; patients are at increased risk for development of lymphoma.

8.5.2 Iatrogenic

8.5.2.1 Medication

Decreased salivary flow with sensation of dry mouth is a frequent side effect of medications, including many commonly prescribed antihypertensives, antidepres-

Fig. 8.10 Cervical dental decay in a patient with Sjögren syndrome.

sants, and antihistamine/decongestants. Medications should be reviewed with this in mind when evaluating patients for complaint of dry mouth.

> **Diagnostic tests**: None. Diagnosis is based on history and review of medications.
> **Biopsy**: No.
> **Treatment**: Discontinue medication if feasible; otherwise symptomatic treatment as described above.
> **Follow-up**: No.

8.5.2.2 Radiation

External beam radiation therapy for head and neck cancer may cause irreversible damage to the salivary glands, particularly the serous acini, with resulting xerostomia that can be quite severe (Fig. 8.11). Patients often

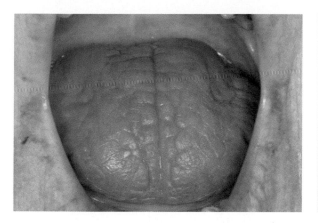

Fig. 8.11 Parched and atrophic tongue with total loss of papillae in a patient following radiation therapy.

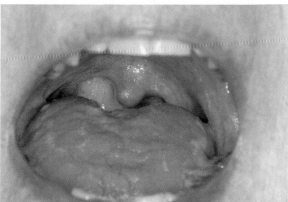

Fig. 8.13 Very thick, ropey, secretions in the oropharynx following radiation therapy. Such lesions can lead to a sensation of choking.

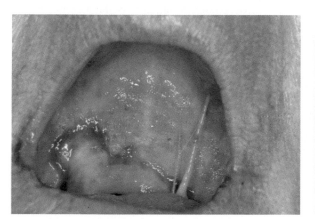

Fig. 8.12 Viscous and adherent secretions in a patient with radiation-induced salivary gland hypofunction.

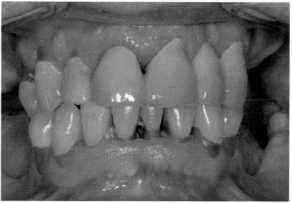

Fig. 8.14 Typical pattern of radiation-associated dental caries affecting the cervical areas.

develop highly viscous secretions that can be difficult to clear from the throat (Figs. 8.12 and 8.13). These patients require close dental follow-up with aggressive preventive maintenance due to the high risk for rampant caries that tends to affect the cervical and root regions of the teeth (Fig. 8.14). Restoration and preservation of teeth is very important given the potential for *osteoradionecrosis* of the jaws following extraction of teeth present in the field of radiation (see Chap. 9).

Treatment with *radioactive iodine* following surgery for thyroid cancer can also result in inflammation and damage to the major salivary glands in a small percentage of patients. Symptoms are usually temporary, unless strictures occur within the ducts resulting in chronic sialadenitis. Sialography, which has now been largely supplanted by computed tomography and is rarely indicated, may be useful in these patients to identify ductal strictures. Treatment of chronic disease is difficult and

often unsatisfactory. Symptoms can sometimes be alleviated with injection of contrast medium during sialography; strictures may be amenable to dilatation via intraoral endoscopic techniques in some cases.

> **Diagnostic tests**: Usually none, as diagnosis is based on a history of radiation therapy and clinical exam. Sialography may be indicated in select situations.
>
> **Biopsy**: No.
>
> **Treatment**: Symptomatic, as discussed above. Cases in which a discrete duct stricture is identified may be amenable to endoscopic dilatation. Pilocarpine or cevimiline may be helpful in cases of external beam irradiation where there is residual functional salivary tissue.
>
> **Follow-up**: As needed.

8.6 Neoplasia

Both benign and malignant lesions arise in the major and minor salivary glands, however, the overall incidence of primary salivary gland cancer is low. Approximately 65–80% of all salivary tumors occur in the parotid gland and the majority of these (about 80%) are benign. Ten to fifteen percent of tumors occur in minor salivary gland tissue with approximately half being malignant. Most minor salivary gland lesions are seen on the posterolateral palate; these may exhibit a bluish hue and be mistaken initially for a mucocele (Fig. 8.15). Approximately 10% of tumors arise in the submandibular gland with up to 40% incidence of malignancy in these lesions. Tumors are very rare in the sublingual gland, but 70–90% of these prove to be malignant.

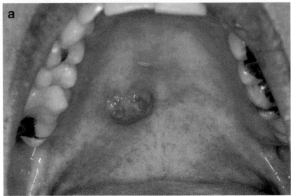

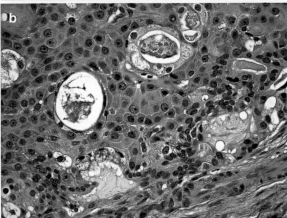

Fig. 8.15 Mucoepidermoid carcinoma of the hard palate. (**a**) The lesion is well defined, exophytic, and reddish purple with focal areas of ulceration. (**b**) Incisional biopsy was interpreted as *low grade* and the lesion was managed with wide excision. Photomicrograph courtesy of Mark Lerman, DMD, Boston, MA.

The majority of salivary gland neoplasms are of epithelial origin, arising from acinar, ductal, or supporting cells. Most present as asymptomatic swellings, however, they can be painful or ulcerated depending on tumor type and location. Paresthesia or facial nerve weakness may indicate neural involvement. Nonepithelial neoplasms, such as lymphoma, hemangiopericytoma, schwannoma, and fibrosarcoma, are much less common but can occur.

8.6.1 Benign Tumors

The *pleomorphic adenoma*, or "benign mixed tumor," is the most common salivary gland neoplasm and occurs in all locations, although is seen most often in the parotid gland. These lesions are painless and slow growing, and are often noted incidentally on exam as a firm mass. Surgical excision is recommended, as they can become quite large and have potential for malignant transformation over time. The lesion should be excised with a margin of surrounding tissue, as opposed to simple enucleation, to minimize recurrence.

The *Warthin tumor*, occurring almost exclusively in the parotid gland, is the second most common salivary neoplasm and may present bilaterally. It is slow growing, asymptomatic, and usually somewhat soft to palpation. Surgical excision is recommended, although malignant transformation is very rare.

8.6.2 Malignant Tumors

The most common malignant salivary tumor is the *mucoepidermoid carcinoma*, which generally presents as a painless swelling in the gland of origin (usually parotid). Treatment and prognosis depends on the location, histologic grade, and stage of the tumor. In general, low-grade lesions exhibit a fairly good prognosis, whereas high-grade tumors can be extremely aggressive and refractory to treatment.

Adenoid cystic carcinoma is seen in the oral cavity arising from minor salivary gland tissue, mainly in the palate. Intraoral lesions are slow growing and may appear ulcerated. This tumor is notorious for its predilection for perineural invasion, which results in pain and a propensity for recurrence. Management is complicated by a high incidence of local recurrence many years after treatment as well as distant metastasis; overall prognosis is poor.

Acinic cell carcinoma is a low-grade salivary malignancy that does not occur very often in the oral cavity, as it affects mainly serous glandular elements. Prognosis is very good in general following surgical resection. *Polymorphous low-grade adenocarcinoma* is another low-grade lesion with good prognosis. It is seen primarily in minor salivary gland tissue and can be found on the palate, lip, and buccal mucosa.

Metastasis of cancer to the salivary glands from another primary site is uncommon. This is seen primarily with skin cancer (mainly squamous cell carcinoma and melanoma) spreading to intraparotid lymph nodes. Attention to examination of the salivary glands in patients with a history of sun exposure who are at risk for skin cancer is therefore important, especially given the recent rise in incidence of skin cancer.

Sources

Baurmash HD, Mucoceles and ranulas. J Oral Maxillofac Surg 2003;61:369–78

Bell RB, Dierks EJ, Horner L, et al. Management and outcome of patients with malignant salivary gland tumors. J Oral Maxillofac Surg 2005;63:917–28

Guggenheimer J, Moore PA. Xerostomia: etiology, recognition and treatment. J Am Dent Assoc 2003;134:61–9

Hinerman RW, Indelicato DJ, Amdur RJ, et al. Cutaneous squamous cell carcinoma metastatic to parotid-area lymph nodes. Laryngoscope 2008;118:1989–96

Mandel L, Liu F. Salivary gland injury resulting from exposure to radioactive iodine: case reports. J Am Dent Assoc 2007;138:1582–7

Madani G, Beale T. Inflammatory conditions of the salivary glands. Semin Ultrasound CT MRI 2006;27:440–51

Mathews S, Kurien B, Scofield R. Oral manifestations of Sjögren's syndrome. J Dent Res 2008;87:308–18

von Bültzingslöwen I, Sollecito TP, Fox PC, et al. Salivary dysfunction associated with systemic diseases: systematic review and clinical management recommendations. Oral Surg Oral Med Oral pathol Oral Radiol Endod 2007;103:S57.e1–15

Shiboski CH, Hidgson TA, Ship JA, et al. Management of salivary hypofunction during and after radiotherapy. Oral Surg Oral Med Oral pathol Oral Radiol Endod 2007;103:S66.e1–19

Chapter 9
Oral Cancer

Summary Oral cancer imposes a significant burden on public health in the USA and many parts of the world. The morbidity of the disease and its treatment can be quite substantial, resulting in disfigurement, pain, impaired speech and swallowing, and overall decreased quality of life. Unfortunately, overall 5-year survival remains approximately 50%, which has not improved significantly over time despite technological advances in treatment. This chapter outlines the epidemiology, major known risk factors, and clinical features of oral malignant and premalignant lesions as well as management guidelines.

Keywords Oral cancer • Squamous cell carcinoma • Carcinogen • Smokeless tobacco • Synergistic effect • Betel • Dyskeratosis congenita • Fanconi anemia • Plummer–Vinson syndrome • Sanguinaria • Exophytic • Tobacco • Alcohol • Fixation • Induration • Verrucous carcinoma • Dysplasia • Carcinoma-in-situ • Cytology • Biopsy • Actinic cheilitis • Leukoplakia • Erythroplakia • Proliferative verrucous leukoplakia • Tobacco pouch keratosis • Oral submucous fibrosis • Lichen planus • Cancer staging • Metastasis • Mucositis • Osteoradionecrosis • Xerostomia • Radiation therapy • Chemotherapy • Hyperbaric oxygen therapy

9.1   Introduction

Oral cancer imposes a significant burden on public health in the USA and many parts of the world. The morbidity of the disease and its treatment can be quite substantial, resulting in disfigurement, pain, impaired speech and swallowing, and overall decreased quality of life. Current research into the molecular biology of carcinogenesis is giving us deeper insight into the etiology and pathogenesis of oral cancer, which will hopefully lead to more effective strategies for diagnosis and treatment in the future. At this point in time, alcohol and tobacco are the two major known causative agents of oral cancer and the majority of head and neck cancer patients consume one or both products. Education and prevention are therefore of high priority in the overall management of this problem.

9.2   Epidemiology

The incidence of oral and oropharyngeal cancer in the USA is approximately 30,000 cases per year, accounting for 2–4% of all cancers diagnosed annually. Worldwide, it ranks as the sixth leading cause of cancer. The vast majority of cancers are epithelial in origin, with *squamous cell carcinoma* (SCCA) being the most common. Unfortunately, overall 5-year survival is only about 50%, which has not improved significantly over time despite technological advances in treatment. Survival is much higher for localized disease, with a survival rate 5 years after treatment of about 80% for patients with early disease versus approximately 20% for those with advanced stage disease. Only about one-third of oral cancer, however, is detected at an early stage, underscoring the importance of early diagnosis. Cancer screening in the community by physicians, nurses, dentists, hygienists, and other healthcare professionals is of critical importance in gaining ground against this disease.

The majority of oral cancer occurs in patients over the age of 40 with the average age at diagnosis between 60 and 65 years. Men are affected more than women by a factor of two, which is presumably related to differences in tobacco usage. This gender gap has been closing steadily over the past 50 years and is likely to continue. The incidence is higher in African-Americans than whites, with African-Americans also exhibiting a higher mortality rate from the disease. Patients diagnosed with oral cancer have an increased incidence of developing additional malignancies (*second primary tumors*) of the upper aerodigestive tract, particularly in smokers who continue the habit following treatment; these patients need to be closely monitored.

9.3 Risk Factors

There are a number of known risk factors for oral SCCA, with tobacco and alcohol being the most notable. Others have been implicated but are not as well characterized. It is important to remember that many cancers arise in the absence of identifiable risk factors and any patient who presents with suspicious signs or symptoms must be fully evaluated.

9.3.1 Tobacco

Tobacco in all forms is a major risk factor for oral SCCA. A large number of carcinogens have been identified in tobacco and its combustion products, the most important of which are polycyclic aromatic hydrocarbons containing benzene, tobacco-specific nitrosamines, and aromatic amines. These compounds result in damage to epithelium in a dose-dependent fashion, with disruption of DNA repair mechanisms and potentially critical genetic mutations leading to malignant transformation. Smokers have about a five- to ten-fold risk of developing oral cancer over nonsmokers. This will decrease by approximately half over a 5-year period if they stop smoking and will reach the risk of a nonsmoker after about 10 years. Cigar and pipe smokers experience a risk profile similar to that of cigarette smokers.

Smokeless tobacco is associated with a lower risk of oral cancer than smoked tobacco, however, it should not be considered "safe" to use nor an acceptable substitute for cigarettes. Risk varies with the composition of the particular product that is used and can be up to fourfold higher than that of a non-user. It is thought that tobacco-specific nitrosamines induce dysplastic changes in the epithelium, which is probably intensified with prolonged surface contact.

9.3.2 Alcohol

Alcohol consumption by itself imparts an increased risk for oral cancer in "moderate to heavy" drinkers; this is variably defined but roughly equivalent to five to eight drinks per day (with one drink containing 1.5 oz or 10–15 gm of alcohol). Importantly, the combined use of alcohol and tobacco produces a *synergistic effect*, in which the presence of one substance enhances the effect of the second. This results in a much greater risk than would be expected by a simple summation of the individual responses. It is thought that ethanol may alter the permeability of the oral mucosa to various substances, including carcinogens, thereby enhancing their penetration into the tissues.

9.3.3 Sun Exposure

Sun exposure is a risk factor for lip cancer due to the cumulative effects of ultraviolet damage. The lower lip is more commonly affected, as it tends to receive relatively more direct exposure to the sun than the upper lip. Sun exposure is not a risk factor for intraoral SCCA or mucosal melanoma.

9.3.4 Betel

Betel products, derived from the nut of the areca palm, are commonly used in parts of the world such as Southeast Asia and the Indian subcontinent, and are believed to be carcinogenic. Preparations usually consist of a mixture of betel nut, betel leaf, tobacco, and slaked lime (calcium hydroxide). Addition of lime enhances the euphoric effect, although it may also potentiate carcinogenicity. Long term use is associated with development of *submucous fibrosis* (see below). Clinicians should be aware that certain immigrant populations to the USA may continue to use these products and should be screened for cancer.

9.3.5 Viral

A number of viruses have been associated with benign and malignant neoplasia of the head and neck. *Epstein-Barr Virus* (EBV) has long been linked to nasopharyngeal carcinoma, Burkitt lymphoma, and other lymphomas. A strain of *human herpesvirus* (HHV-8) is believed to be associated with development of Kaposi sarcoma (see Chap. 6) in HIV-infected patients. *Human papillomavirus* (HPV) is well known to cause benign proliferative epithelial lesions throughout the head and neck region, including *squamous papilloma* and *condylomata* (see Chap. 7). More recently, high-risk strains of HPV (particularly 16 and 18; associated with cancer of the uterine cervix) have been identified in tumors of the posterior oral cavity/oropharynx. The exact nature of viral involvement with initiation or progression of malignancy in these cases in not yet clear and speculation on the potential impact of the newly introduced HPV vaccine for oral cancer is premature. This is currently an active area of research that will hopefully produce valuable information in the near future.

9.3.6 Immunosuppression

Immunosuppressed individuals are at increased risk for malignancy in the oral cavity and elsewhere in the body. HIV-infected patients in particular can develop oral SCCA, Kaposi sarcoma, and non-Hodgkin lymphoma. Transplant patients are at risk for multiple malignancies including lip and mouth cancer. Patients with *dyskeratosis congenita*, which is a very rare inherited condition of progressive bone marrow failure leading to aplastic anemia, present with skin hyperpigmentation, dystrophic nail changes, and *leukoplakia* (see below). Leukoplakic lesions in these patients exhibit a particularly high risk of malignant transformation (Fig. 9.1). Patients with *Fanconi anemia*, a similarly rare bone marrow failure syndrome, are also at high risk for developing oral SCCA.

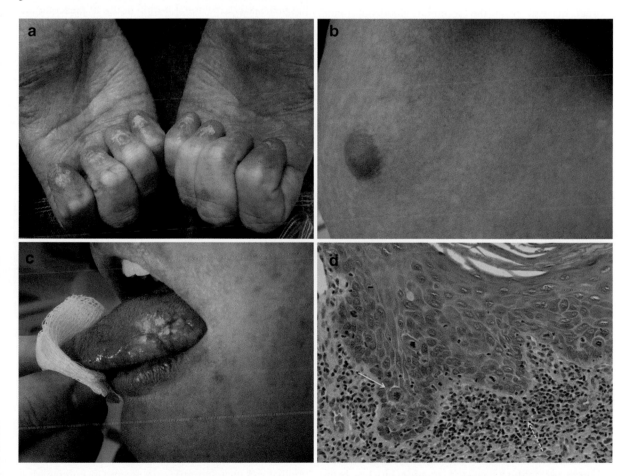

Fig. 9.1 Dyskeratosis congenita. (**a**) Dystrophic nails and leathery, cracked palms. (**b**) Hypo- and hyperpigmentation of the skin. (**c**) Diffuse lateral tongue leukoplakia. (**d**) Biopsy of the tongue demonstrated dysplasia with maturational disarray and large mitotic figures (*solid arrow*) with an inflammatory infiltrate (*broken arrow*). Reprinted from Treister et al. (2004), with permission from Elsevier.

9.3.7 Nutrition

Nutritional factors, such as vitamin and mineral deficiencies, are thought to play some role in carcinogenesis, although no specific causative pathway has been elicited. This is possibly related to loss of an antioxidant mechanism and formation of damaging free radicals. Patients with *Plummer–Vinson syndrome*, which is a rare condition presenting with dysphagia, esophageal webs, and iron deficiency anemia in middle-aged women, are thought to be at increased risk for esophageal and oral carcinoma.

9.3.8 Sanguinaria

Extract derived from the common bloodroot plant *Sanguinaria canadensis*, has been used commercially in oral rinses and toothpaste as an antibacterial agent to reduce plaque and gingivitis. It has been linked to development of leukoplakia occurring particularly in the region of the maxillary vestibule. Monitoring of patients who have used these products is advised, although the risk of malignant change in these lesions is unclear and is probably not high. The main commercial marketer in the USA has removed sanguinaria from its products; however, dentrifices containing this herbal supplement are still available and their use should be discouraged.

9.3.9 Other

Marijuana smoking has been implicated as a potential risk factor for oral cancer; however, this has not been clearly substantiated to date. *Hyperplastic candidiasis* (see Chap. 7) may be associated with premalignant lesions, as invasion of fungal elements has been demonstrated in some thick or nodular leukoplakias, however, this relationship is unclear with respect to development of cancer. Historically, *syphilis* has been linked to an increased incidence of tongue cancer, although no definite causative relationship has been established.

9.4 High-Risk Sites

9.4.1 Tongue

The tongue is the most common location for oral cancer in the USA, with more than half of lesions presenting on the *oral tongue*, and the remainder occurring in the *tongue base*. In the oral cavity proper, lesions are most frequently seen on the lateral and ventral surfaces, and these areas are considered particularly high-risk sites. The overall incidence of tongue cancer has increased somewhat over the last 20 years, with some concern for increasing frequency at this site in patients under the age of 40 who do not have a history of tobacco use or other known risk factors. In general, malignancies of the tongue base tend to be more advanced at the time of diagnosis, with up to three-fourths already exhibiting metastasis to regional lymph nodes at presentation. This may be partly due to greater difficulty in visualizing and palpating the area on examination, causing these lesions to remain "hidden" longer.

9.4.2 Lip

The vermillion of the lip is the second most common site for oral cancer, and this has been decreasing in incidence over time. The majority of labial carcinomas occur on the lower lip, more frequently in men than women. Ultraviolet radiation exposure is the major risk factor for this area, and increased occupational and/or recreational sun exposure in men is thought to account for the gender difference. Use of lipstick and other topical protectants may also contribute to the lower incidence in women. Cancer can arise in pipe smokers where the pipestem contacts the lip repeatedly over a long period of time.

Lip cancers in general are diagnosed at an early stage due to their relatively high visibility, and can usually be treated surgically with an overall 5-year survival rate of 90%. Poorer prognosis is associated with lesions on the upper lip or commissure region. From an epidemiologic standpoint, lip cancers are often grouped with skin cancers, as they have a distinctive risk factor profile and prognosis compared to intraoral mucosal carcinomas.

9.4.3 Floor of Mouth

Pooling of secretions in the floor of mouth is thought to potentiate contact of carcinogens with the tissues. In addition, the very thin, nonkeratinized mucosa in this area may provide less of a barrier for penetration of toxic substances than might be found in other parts of the oral cavity. Cancers in this area can be quite aggressive and present with early lymph node involvement due to the rich lymphatic supply.

9.5 Signs and Symptoms

9.5.1 Squamous Cell Carcinoma

The clinical presentation of oral SCCA is quite varied, and necessitates a high level of awareness and vigilance during the oral examination. Lesions may appear flat (*macular*; Fig. 9.2), raised (*plaque-like*; Fig. 9.3), *exophytic* (growing outward; Fig. 9.4), or *ulcerated* (showing surface erosion; Figs. 9.5 and 9.6). The surface texture can range from smooth to irregular. *Induration* (firmness or hardness; Fig. 9.7) and *fixation* (immobility or palpable adherence to underlying structures) indicate infiltration of cancer cells into deeper tissues. These lesions have the potential for local bone destruction and nerve invasion as well as more distant spread via the lymphatics and bloodstream. Pain is a worrisome symptom, although lack of pain does not exclude malignancy.

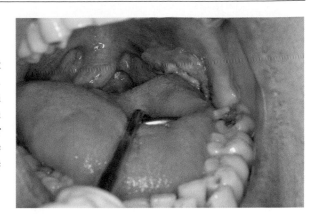

Fig. 9.3 Squamous cell carcinoma of the left soft palate presenting as an exophytic mass with central ulceration.

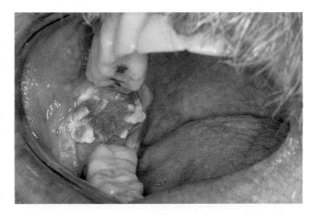

Fig. 9.4 Large exophytic squamous cell carcinoma of the buccal mucosa with heavy keratinization and induration.

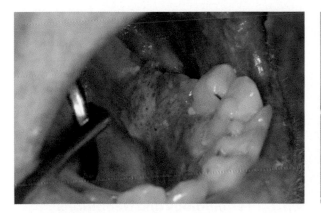

Fig. 9.2 Squamous cell carcinoma of the mandibular ridge with erythroleukoplakia and focal areas of ulceration. This patient developed multifocal involvement, suggestive of a *field cancerization* effect.

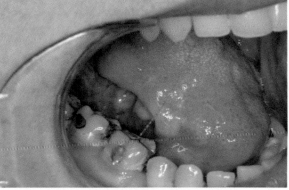

Fig. 9.5 Large squamous cell carcinoma of the right lateral tongue with ulceration and induration.

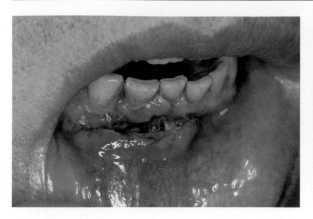

Fig. 9.6 Squamous cell carcinoma of the mandibular labial vestibule presenting as a clefted, indurated mass with central ulceration and necrosis.

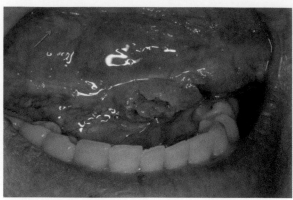

Fig. 9.8 Papillary verruciform squamous cell carcinoma of the ventral tongue. This lesion developed in the context of leukoplakic changes that can be partly seen on the superior aspect of the lateral tongue (*arrow*).

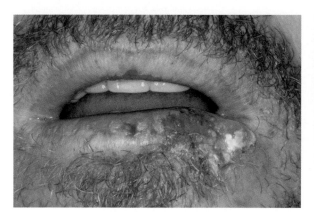

Fig. 9.7 Squamous cell carcinoma of the left lower lip with crusting, ulceration, and induration.

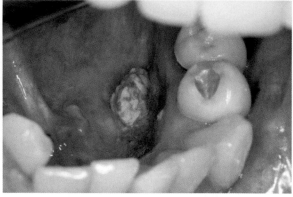

Fig. 9.9 Verrucous carcinoma of the floor of the mouth with surrounding erythroleukoplakia.

Any nonhealing ulcer or extraction socket, as well as any white or red patch that cannot be rubbed off or induced to resolve, should be biopsied. The following can all be warning signs for cancer: difficulty or pain with chewing or swallowing (*dysphagia, odynophagia*), ear pain (*otalgia*), limitation of mouth opening (*trismus*), alteration of speech (*dysarthria*), alteration of sensation such as numbness or tingling (*paresthesia*), cervical lymph node enlargement (*adenopathy*), tooth mobility, or change in the fit of a denture.

9.5.2 Verrucous Carcinoma

Verrucous carcinoma is a low-grade variant of SCCA with a distinctive exophytic and papillary, or warty, appearance (Fig. 9.8). Heavy keratinization causes a typically whitish or gray color (Fig. 9.9); common sites are the buccal mucosa, gingiva, and vestibule. The prognosis is usually more favorable than that of conventional SCCA due to its slow growth, high degree of differentiation, and minimal propensity for metastasis. Treatment consists of local surgical excision without use of radiation or chemotherapy.

9.6 Histopathology

9.6.1 Terminology and Definitions

Epithelial *dysplasia* represents a disruption of the normal orderly growth and maturation process of oral mucosa, which may then progress to *carcinoma in situ* or *invasive carcinoma*. Normally, cell division occurs in the deep *basal layer* of the epithelium (see Chap. 1), which is separated from the underlying connective tissue by a *basement membrane*. New cells migrate upward through the layers of epithelium to replace those that are shed regularly from the surface. Cell maturation and differentiation take place in the process, with mature cells ultimately acquiring their flattened (*squamoid*) shape and ability to make keratin. Keratin production and deposition occurs only in the superficial layers of keratinized tissues. The entire process of epithelial regeneration and turnover is well organized and regulated, with distinct maturational layers (*stratification*) visible histologically (Fig. 9.10).

Cell alteration and *atypia* are seen in dysplastic epithelium, with evidence of abnormal cell division, hyperplasia of the basal cell layer, cell crowding, and loss of the usual stratification pattern (Fig. 9.11). Cell maturation is disordered, with appearance of keratin producing cells or clumps of keratin (*keratin pearls*) in the deeper layers and immature cells more superficially (Fig. 9.12). Dysplasia is a histological diagnosis, and the severity is determined according to proportion of epithelium that exhibits these abnormal features.

Mild dysplasia involves the deeper layers only, generally estimated at no more than 1/3 of the total thickness of the epithelium. *Severe dysplasia* involves the entire thickness of epithelium without disruption of the basement membrane, and is considered equivalent to *carcinoma in situ*. Once the barrier basement membrane between epithelium and connective tissue has been breached by abnormal cells, the lesion is labeled *invasive carcinoma* and possesses the potential for spread (*metastasis*) through the lymphatic or vascular systems (Fig. 9.12). Findings may be reversible in the early stages in some cases if the inciting cause can be identified and eliminated.

9.6.2 Biopsy Considerations

To adequately diagnose invasive carcinoma or determine the degree of dysplasia present, the biopsy specimen must include the full thickness of epithelium with adjacent basement membrane and connective tissue interface. This is obtained by either *incisional* or *excisional biopsy* (see Chap. 3). In general, small lesions are excised fully via excisional biopsy if possible. Incisional biopsy is preferred for larger lesions in order to initially establish the diagnosis and facilitate treatment planning, as a subsequent major resection may be required in conjunction with other treatment modalities.

Exfoliative cytology and brush biopsy techniques (see Chap. 3) can be useful for detecting abnormal appearing cells in a specimen. However, as only individual cells are obtained, these tests do not provide information regarding

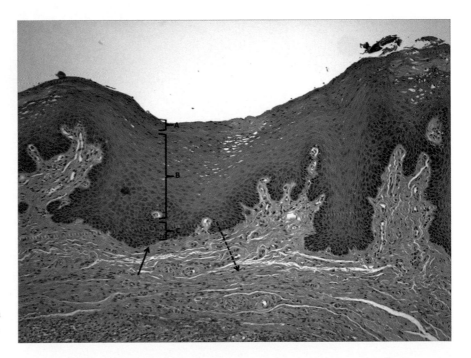

Fig. 9.10 Histology of normal keratinized oral mucosa showing the keratin (**a**), spinous (**b**), and basal (**c**) layers, basement membrane (*solid arrow*), and underlying connective tissue (*broken arrow*). Photomicrograph courtesy of Mark Lerman, DMD, Boston, MA.

Fig. 9.11 Progression of cellular atypia and dysplasia to invasive squamous cell carcinoma: (**a**) mild dysplasia, (**b**) moderate dysplasia, (**c**) severe dysplasia (carcinoma in situ), and (**d**) invasive carcinoma; note breach of basement membrane.

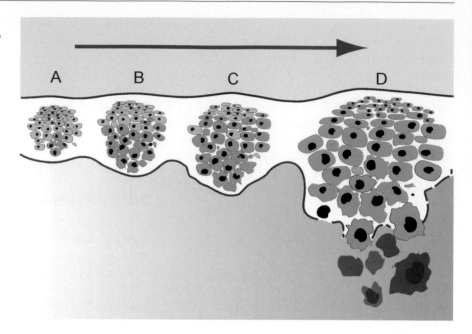

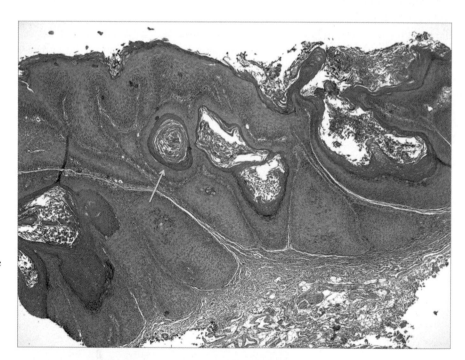

Fig. 9.12 Squamous cell carcinoma histopathology demonstrating dysplastic surface epithelium and invasive tumor islands with keratin pearl formation (*arrow*). Photomicrograph courtesy of Mark Lerman, DMD, Boston, MA.

epithelial architecture or basement membrane integrity. Therefore, the pathologist cannot make a determination regarding dysplasia or carcinoma. These methods may help to guide the practitioner in deciding whether formal biopsy should be performed, but clinical judgment in favor of biopsy should prevail if any suspicion for malignancy remains. *Vital stains*, such as toluidine blue, which bind to DNA and indicate areas of high cell turnover, can also be used as adjuncts for biopsy and monitoring of suspicious lesions.

9.7 Premalignant Lesions

The term premalignant, or "precancerous," implies that there is a known potential for the lesion to transform into malignancy at a rate high enough to warrant pre-emptive action or close observation. As there is no way to predict whether a given lesion will undergo malignant change in a particular individual, a high level of vigilance is necessary.

9.7.1 Actinic Cheilitis (Sailor's lip; Solar cheilitis)

This is a type of *actinic keratosis* which classically occurs on the lower lip and is directly related to long-term sun exposure. It is most frequently seen in white males over age 40. The vermilion appears atrophic and pale, with a glossy surface and loss of demarcation at the vermilion border. With progression, fissuring and ulceration can occur along with crusting or scaling (Fig. 9.13). Epithelial atrophy and elastosis are seen histologically and these changes are irreversible. Areas of persistent ulceration should be biopsied due to a 6–10% rate of malignant transformation. Treatment of malignancy is primarily surgical; however, a trial of topical chemotherapy with 5-fluorouracil can be used with early lesions. Prophylactic laser ablation or vermillionectomy may be performed in cases where malignant transformation has not yet occurred. Close long-term follow-up is indicated, as these patients are at risk for additional cancers associated with solar damage.

9.7.2 Leukoplakia

The term leukoplakia is derived from Greek, meaning literally a "white patch," and is defined by the World Health Organization as a white plaque that cannot be rubbed off or clinically identified as another named entity (such as described in Chap. 4). It is therefore strictly a *clinical* label rather than a *histological* diagnosis. These lesions should be biopsied, after which a more definitive diagnosis can be assigned. Most prove to be benign (usually hyperkeratosis or chronic inflammation), however, up to 20% may exhibit histological changes consistent with dysplasia or carcinoma. They should therefore be regarded with suspicion until proven otherwise, particularly if occurring in a high-risk site such as the ventral or lateral tongue or floor of mouth. The clinical appearance is extremely variable with respect to size, shape, thickness, and homogeneity of color (Figs. 9.14–9.19). They are usually asymptomatic.

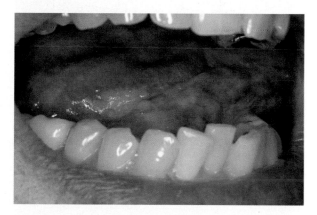

Fig. 9.14 Well-defined, smooth, and homogeneous leukoplakia of the right lateroventral tongue.

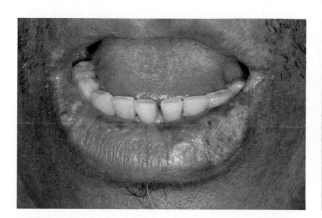

Fig. 9.13 Actinic cheilitis of the lower lip showing crusting, atrophic changes, and loss of vermillion border definition.

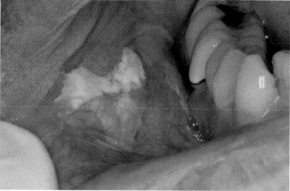

Fig. 9.15 Extensive leukoplakia of the right buccal mucosa with homogenous thin and thick areas extending to the vestibule.

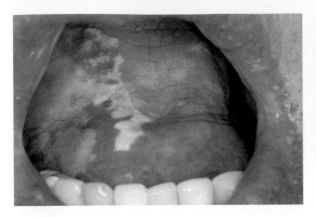

Fig. 9.16 Proliferative leukoplakia involving most of the tongue dorsum, with associated atrophy and depapillation.

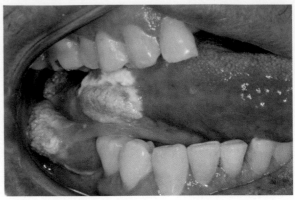

Fig. 9.19 Prominent multifocal, mass-like verrucous leukoplakia of the right lateral tongue in an HIV-positive patient.

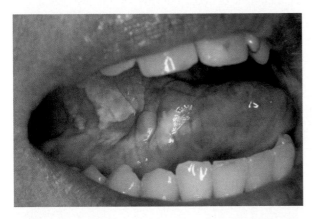

Fig. 9.17 Leukoplakia of the right lateral tongue in a patient previously treated for squamous cell carcinoma of the tongue.

9.7.3   Proliferative Verrucous Leukoplakia

Proliferative verrucous leukoplakia (PVL) is an uncommon but specific type of leukoplakia that is known for a very high rate of malignant change. It is typically thick and exophytic in appearance, although may appear flat in the early stages (Fig. 9.20). Lesions often develop on the buccal mucosa and gingiva; this is in contrast to conventional leukoplakia which is more commonly seen on the ventral/lateral tongue and floor of mouth. There is an unusual predisposition for women over the age of 50 for unknown reasons. Specific risk factors have not been identified, and tobacco use does not appear to be related. It is generally slowly progressive and often multifocal. The treatment of choice is surgical resection, although the extensive and "creeping" nature of these lesions can make definitive therapy extremely challenging. The recurrence rate is high and patients with PVL must be monitored closely.

9.7.4   Tobacco Pouch Keratosis

Tobacco pouch keratosis, also referred to as *snuff dipper's keratosis*, is a unique form of leukoplakia related to the direct effect of smokeless tobacco on the oral mucosa. Lesions occur at the site of contact, which is usually in the mandibular anterior labial vestibule or more posteriorly in the buccal vestibule. The mucosa is gray to whitish in color and wrinkled, and there may

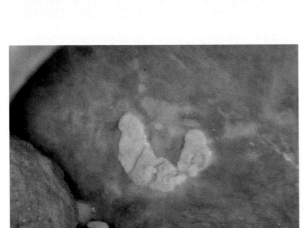

Fig. 9.18 Thick verrucous leukoplakia of the left buccal mucosa in the setting of extensive mucosal changes that have a slightly *lichenoid* appearance. Photograph courtesy of Sook-Bin Woo, DMD, DMSc, Boston, MA.

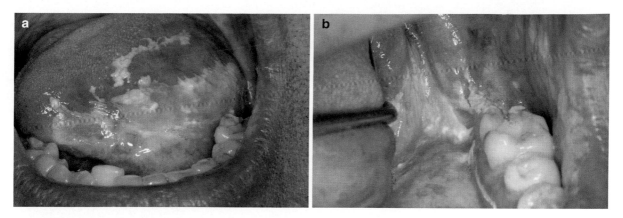

Fig. 9.20 Proliferative verrucous leukoplakia. (a) Extensive involvement of the tongue and (b) floor of mouth with a thick, wrinkled appearance. Photographs courtesy of Sook-Bin Woo, DMD, MMSc, Boston, MA.

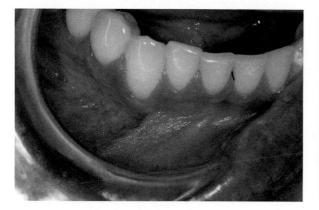

Fig. 9.21 Smokeless tobacco keratosis with thickened, corrugated appearing mucosa in the area where the tobacco is placed.

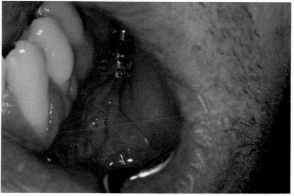

Fig. 9.22 Smokeless tobacco keratosis with deeply wrinkled and fissured appearance.

be an associated pouch-like depression secondary to stretching of the tissue from the mass of tobacco (Figs. 9.21 and 9.22). The lesion becomes increasingly white over time, as well as more leathery or nodular in texture. The neighboring gingiva is commonly inflamed or receded. The risk of malignant transformation is less than that of conventional leukoplakia, and most lesions will resolve several weeks after use of the product is discontinued. Lesions that show ulceration or erythema or that persist despite tobacco cessation, must be biopsied.

betel products and is seen mainly in areas of the world where this practice is endemic. Development of this condition may also be influenced by nutritional and/or genetic factors. Mucosal stiffening occurs over time with formation of fibrotic bands, particularly in the buccal region and soft palate, with gradual onset of trismus (Fig. 9.23). This is progressive and irreversible, with a reported malignant transformation rate ranging from 4% to 13%. Treatment consists of local steroid injection and surgical disruption (*lysis*) of fibrous bands, however, outcomes are generally poor.

9.7.5 Oral Submucous Fibrosis

This represents chronic inflammation with atrophy and fibrosis of the oral mucosa secondary to habitual use of

9.7.6 Erythroplakia

Erythroplakia is derived from Greek, meaning "flat red area," and is a clinically descriptive term without specific

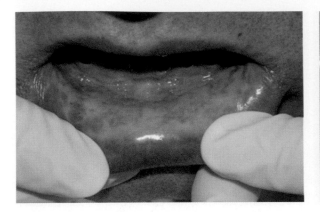

Fig. 9.23 Submucous fibrosis of the lower labial mucosa with loss of vestibule depth in a user of betel product. Photograph courtesy of Ross Kerr, DDS, MSD, New York, NY.

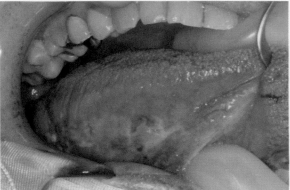

Fig. 9.24 Erythroleukoplakia of the right lateral tongue.

histologic definition. Lesions frequently exhibit a bright red, velvety appearance and are usually asymptomatic. The incidence of severe dysplasia or carcinoma in these lesions is very high (80–90%), and biopsy is mandatory. Areas of erythroplakia may also coexist with leukoplakia in so-called "mixed" or "speckled" lesions (*erythroleukoplakia*; Figs. 9.24–9.26). Care must be taken to obtain a representative biopsy specimen in such cases, with sampling of multiple areas within the lesion, as carcinoma may be present only focally.

9.7.7 Oral Lichen Planus

Development of cancer within an existing area of lichen planus (see Chap. 5) has long been a topic of controversy and no definite answer is available. Whether the two entities arise coincidentally or the atrophic epithelium seen in the erosive/ulcerative form of lichen planus is rendered more susceptible to carcinogens is unclear. Common wisdom dictates that patients with lichen planus be monitored regularly, with biopsy of any areas that are changing or otherwise appear suspicious.

9.8 Cancer Staging

Staging, or defining the extent of cancer, is important with respect to treatment planning and determination of prognosis. Patients in whom cancer is diagnosed at an early stage are generally expected to fare better, and

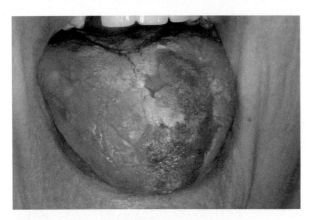

Fig. 9.25 Extensive erythroleukoplakia of the tongue dorsum that initially demonstrated inflammation without dysplasia on biopsy but subsequently transformed to squamous cell carcinoma.

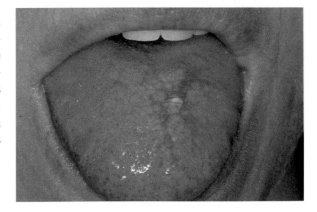

Fig. 9.26 Erythroleukoplakia of the tongue dorsum with thick plaque-like area of leukoplakia.

may require less aggressive therapy than patients with more advanced disease. Accurate staging, with consistent use of accepted and uniform terminology, is also

Table 9.1   TNM classification for oral cancer

Primary tumor (T)	T_x	Primary tumor cannot be assessed
	T_0	No evidence of primary tumor
	T_{is}	Carcinoma in situ
	T_1	Tumor ≤2 cm in greatest dimension
	T_2	Tumor >2 cm in greatest dimension but ≤4 cm
	T_3	Tumor >4 cm
	T_4	Tumor invades deep or adjacent structures *(further subdivided into T4a and T4b)*
Regional lymph nodes (N)	N_x	Lymph nodes cannot be assessed
	N_0	No lymph node metastasis
	N_1	Metastasis in a single ipsilateral lymph node measuring ≤3 cm in greatest dimension
	N_{2a}	Metastasis in a single ipsilateral node measuring >3 cm but ≤6 cm
	N_{2b}	Metastasis in multiple ipsilateral nodes, none measuring >6 cm
	N_{2c}	Metastasis in bilateral or contralateral nodes, none >6 cm
	N_3	Metastasis in a node >6 cm
Distant metastasis (M)	M_x	Distant metastasis cannot be assessed
	M_0	No distant metastasis
	M_1	Distant metastasis present

Table 9.2   Stage groupings for oral cancer

Stage	TNM classification
0	$T_{is} N_0 M_0$
I	$T_1 N_0 M_0$
II	$T_2 N_0 M_0$
III	$T_3 N_0 M_0$
	$T_{1-3} N_1 M_0$
IV(further subdivided into IVA,IVB, and IVC)	$T_4 N_0 M_0$
	$T_4 N_1 M_0$
	$T_{any} N_{2-3} M_0$
	$T_{any} N_{any} M_1$

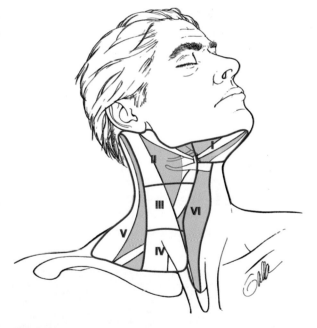

Fig. 9.27 Cervical lymph node groups by levels. (Reprinted with permission from Janfaza (2001); Lippincott Williams and Wilkins).

necessary to evaluate outcomes of cancer therapy and compare data across different populations.

The staging system for head and neck cancer that is currently in use follows the American Joint Committee on Cancer (AJCC) cancer staging manual, which was most recently revised in 2002 (6th edition). This is based on the clinically determined anatomic extent of the primary tumor and tumor spread. It does not take into account histological or biological features of the lesion. It is referred to as the "TNM system," describing tumor size (T), lymph node involvement (N), and metastasis to distant sites (M). These three parameters taken together determine the stage of disease, with stage IV being the most advanced and carrying the worst prognosis (Tables 9.1 and 9.2).

Oral SCCA metastasizes primarily through the lymphatic system to regional cervical lymph nodes in a relatively predictable pattern. The neck is anatomically divided into "levels," which helps to define the extent of lymph node involvement and guide treatment planning (Fig. 9.27). The presence of lymph node involvement at the time of diagnosis dramatically worsens the patient's prognosis. Lymphatic drainage from oral cavity sites (see Chap. 1) are primarily to level I (submental, submandibular) and level II (upper jugular) lymph nodes, however, other levels can be involved. Suspicious clinical signs include nontender node enlargement, very firm or hard consistency of the node on palpation, and fixation (immobility). Fixation indicates penetration of cancer through the lymph node capsule with spread and adherence of tumor to adjacent tissues (*extracapsular extension*). In contrast, normal lymph nodes responding to an inflammatory insult (*reactive nodes*) are generally enlarged but tender, rubbery in consistency, and mobile.

Metastasis of cancer cells through the bloodstream results in spread to more distant tissues (*distant metastasis*), such as the brain and lungs. Presence of distant metastasis (M1 designation in the TNM system) indicates advanced disease and is classified as stage IV.

9.9 Treatment

Treatment is largely determined by location and extent of disease following full workup and staging. Other factors are taken into consideration, including general health and nutritional status of the patient with respect to their ability to tolerate (or wish to pursue) various treatment options. Treatment planning is now frequently carried out in a multidisciplinary fashion, involving a team of practitioners from a range of specialty areas, including surgery (otolaryngology/head and neck or oral/maxillofacial), radiation oncology, medical oncology, radiology, speech/swallowing pathology, and dentistry. Ancillary and support services are important to help the patient and family through a potentially long, difficult, and often debilitating course of therapy.

Lip cancer, particularly of the lower lip, generally responds very well to surgical excision with a 5-year survival rate of greater than 90%. Surgical resection is also the primary treatment modality for intraoral SCCA, with 5-year survival varying widely depending on the extent and location of disease. Surgical removal of regional lymph nodes is indicated when there is evidence of lymph node involvement at the time of diagnosis or significant risk for spread to the lymph nodes. Postoperative radiation therapy is recommended for advanced stage cancers in which there is high risk for recurrent disease or metastasis. For tumors located more posteriorly, such as base of tongue, combined treatment with radiation and chemotherapy may be chosen as the primary treatment modality with surgery reserved as a secondary option if needed.

All treatment modalities are associated with potentially unpleasant or debilitating side effects. Surgery can result in disfigurement and sensory changes of the mucosa as well as functional deficits in speech, swallowing, and breathing (Figs. 9.28–9.30). These can lead to poor nutritional intake and social isolation. Radiation therapy causes both acute and chronic side effects; mucositis (Fig. 9.31) and reddening of the skin in the field of radiation are common acute effects. The major late effects include xerostomia (see Chap. 6), hypothyroidism, trismus, and *osteoradionecrosis* (ORN) of the jaws (Fig. 9.32). Radiation-induced xerostomia can lead to rampant severe caries that can be quite problematic to treat and aggressive preventive dental care is necessary in these patients (see Chap. 8). ORN is a potentially devastating complication of radiation therapy that is often precipitated by trauma to irradiated

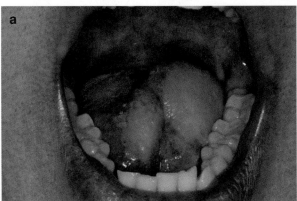
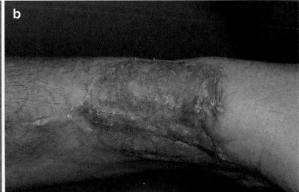

Fig. 9.28 Hemiglossectomy with surgical reconstruction using a free-tissue transfer graft from the forearm. (**a**) The left side of the tongue has a thick, pale, "skin-like" appearance compared with the mucosa on the right. (**b**) Appearance of the healing graft harvest site.

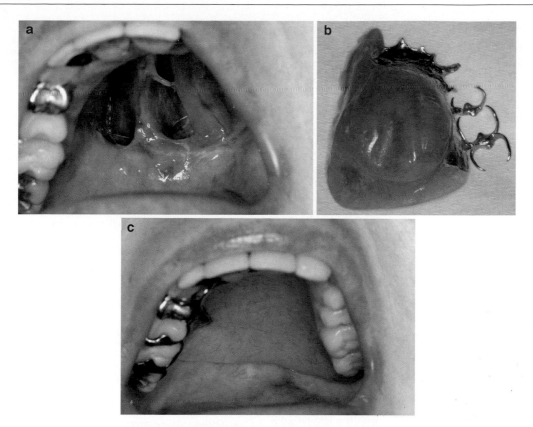

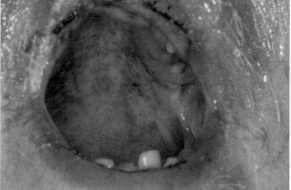

Fig. 9.29 Partial maxillectomy surgical defect functionally restored with a prosthesis. (**a**) Anatomical defect in the hard palate. (**b**) Maxillary prosthesis (obturator) used to seal the opening from the oral cavity into the nasal cavity and maxillary sinus. (**c**) Prosthesis in place allowing patient to eat, swallow, and speak comfortably.

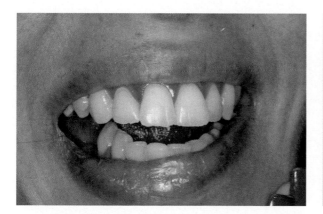

Fig. 9.30 22 year-old female with severe trismus following radiation therapy for nasopharyngeal carcinoma. This represents the patient's maximum opening.

Fig. 9.31 Typical radiation mucositis of the palate with irregularly shaped ulcer and associated erythema. There is also ulceration of the upper labial mucosa.

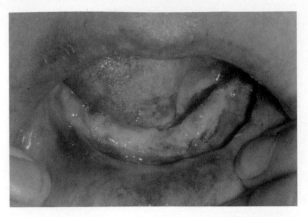

Fig. 9.32 Osteoradionecrosis of the mandible. The necrotic bone appears yellow and ragged with edematous surrounding gingiva. Note the large amalgam tattoo in the right labial mucosa. Photograph courtesy of Stephen Sonis, DMD, DMSc, Boston, MA.

bone or extraction of teeth within the field of radiation. Fibrosis and compromised blood supply secondary to radiation can lead to poor wound healing and bone necrosis. Surgical debridement and hyperbaric oxygen (used to encourage wound healing through increased oxygen tension and stimulation of vascular proliferation) may be required for treatment for this problem.

Treatment of oral cancer remains challenging despite best efforts, with poor overall survival rates for advanced disease. Research in the field is active, however, and the future will hopefully bring new advances. In the meantime, the clinician should be aware that the best chance for cure lies in detection and treatment of disease in the earliest stages.

Sources

Aldington S, Harwood M, Cox B, et al. Cannabis use and cancer of the head and neck: case-control study. Otolaryngol Head Neck Surg 2008;138:374–80

Atkinson JC, Harvey KE, Domingo DL, et al. Oral and dental phenotype of dyskeratosis congenita. Oral Dis 2008;14: 419–27

Brennan M, Migliorati CA, Lockhart PB, et al. Management of oral epithelial dysplasia: a review. Oral Surg Oral Med Oral Pathol Oral Radiol Endod 2007;103;S19.e1–12

Cabay RJ, Morton TH, Epstein JB. Proliferative verrucous leukoplakia and its progression to oral carcinoma: a review of the literature. J Oral Pathol Med 2007;36:255–61

Cavalcante A, Anbinder A, Carvalho Y. Actinic cheilitis: clinical and histological features. J Oral Maxillofac Surg 2008;66: 498–503

D'Souza G, Kreimer, A, Viscidi R, et al. Case-control study of human papillomavirus and oropharyngeal cancer. N Engl J Med 2007; 356:1944–56

Eversole LR, Eversole GM, Kopcik J. Sanguinaria-associated oral leukoplakia. Oral Surg Oral Med Oral Pathol Oral Radiol Endod 2000;89:455–64

Greene FL, Page DL, Pleming ID, et al. eds. AJCC Cancer Staging Manual. 6th ed. New York, NY: Springer, 2002

Haddad R, Annino D, Tishler RB. Multidisciplinary approach to cancer treatment: focus on head and neck cancer. Dent Clin North Am 2008;52:1–17

Haddad R, Shin D. Recent advances in head and neck cancer. N Engl J Med 2008;359:1143–54

Janfaza P. Surgical anatomy of the head and neck. Hagerstown, MD: Lippincott Williams and Wilkins, 2001

Johnson NW, Bain CA, et al. Tobacco and oral disease. Br Dent J 2000;189:200–6

Lodi G, Sardella A, Bez C. Interventions for treating leukoplakia. Cochrane Database Syst Rev 2006;18:CD001829

Maserejian NN, Joshipura KJ, Rosner BA, et al. Prospective study of alcohol consumption and risk of oral premalignant lesions in men. Cancer Epidemiol Biomarkers Prev 2006;15:774–81

Morse DE, Psoter WJ, Cleveland D, et al. Smoking and drinking in relation to oral cancer and oral epithelial dysplasia. Cancer Causes Control 2007;18:919–29

Munoz AA, Haddad RI, Woo SB, et al. Behavior of oral squamous cell carcinoma in subjects with prior lichen planus. Otolaryngol Head Neck Surg 2007;136:401–4

Rodrigo JP, Suarez C, Shaha AR. New molecular diagnostic methods in head and neck cancer. Head Neck 2005;27:995–1003

Tilakaratne WM, Klinikowski MF, Saku T, et al. Oral submucous fibrosis: a review of aetiology and pathogenesis. Oral Oncol 2006;42:561–8

Treister NS, Lehmann L, Cherrick I, et al. Dyskeratosis congenita vs. chronic graft versus host disease: report of a case and a review of the literature. Oral Surg Oral Med Oral Pathol Oral Radiol Endod 2004; 98:566–71

Van der Waal I. Potentially malignant disorders of the oral and oropharyngeal mucosa; terminology, classification, and present concepts of management. Oral Oncol 2008;45(4–5):317–23

Warnakulasuriya S, Reibel J, Boquot J, et al. Oral epithelial dysplasia classification systems: predictive value, utility, weakness, and scope for improvement. J Oral Pathol Med 2008;37:127–33

Chapter 10
Orofacial Pain Conditions

Summary Orofacial pain is a common symptom that causes significant morbidity. The majority of orofacial pain disorders can be classified as *odontogenic, myofascial, temporomandibular joint-related*, and *neuropathic*. A careful history accompanied by a comprehensive examination in most cases is sufficient to determine the correct diagnosis, although laboratory tests and imaging studies may be indicated. Careful explanation of the diagnosis and establishment of realistic treatment goals are critically important for successful outcomes. This chapter provides a rational approach to the evaluation, diagnosis, and management of patients with orofacial pain.

Keywords Nociceptive • Allodynia • Neuropathic pain • Dysesthesia • Odontogenic pain • Referred pain • Temporomandibular joint pain • Arthralgia • Myofascial pain disorder • Parafunctional activity • Bruxism • Trigger point • Crepitus • Atypical facial pain • Persistent idiopathic facial pain • Atypical odontalgia • Trigeminal neuralgia • Glossopharyngeal neuralgia • Occipital neuralgia • Burning mouth syndrome • Stomatodynia

10.1 Introduction

Pain is defined as an unpleasant sensory and emotional experience that is associated with actual or potential tissue damage, or described in such terms even in the absence of any obvious damage. *Nociceptive pain*, on the one hand, is caused by actual tissue injury and inflammation, such as seen with pulpal involvement of a tooth secondary to dental caries, and is an important physiological protective mechanism. *Neuropathic pain*, on the other hand, is caused by dysfunction of the central and/or peripheral nervous system in the absence of active injury or inflammation, such as *post-herpetic neuralgia*, that results in neurosensory signs and symptoms. The term *dysesthesia* refers to an unpleasant sensation, such as "burning," that is either spontaneous or evoked. *Allodynia* is used to describe pain caused by a stimulus that would not normally induce pain, such as light touch or chewing. Importantly, management varies greatly depending on the type, duration, and quality of pain.

Orofacial pain is a common symptom that causes significant morbidity. Diagnosis requires a careful history and examination. As the trigeminal nerve supplies a great deal of sensory and motor innervation to the face and jaws, it is not surprising that branches of this nerve are most commonly responsible for orofacial pain conditions. Cranial nerves VII, IX, X, and XII can also be involved. Although there are many different potential causes of pain in the head and neck region, the vast majority of cases fall into the following categories based on the structures affected: *odontogenic, myofascial, temporomandibular joint, neuropathic*, and *headache* (Table 10.1). Odontogenic pain is reviewed briefly later, as it is discussed in the context of odontogenic infection in Chap. 7. Headache conditions, which often have an underlying vascular and/or muscular etiology, are not included in this discussion. When signs or symptoms suggestive of a central lesion or tumor are present, appropriate testing and consultations should be obtained.

An individual's perception of pain is highly subjective and is influenced by the underlying cause, which may not be clinically evident, as well as emotional and psychological factors. Key components of the history include: the timing, duration, quality, and intensity of pain; modifiers that make the pain better or worse;

J.M. Bruch and N.S. Treister, *Clinical Oral Medicine and Pathology*,
DOI 10.1007/978-1-60327-520-0_10, © Humana Press, a part of Springer Science+Business Media, LLC 2010

Table 10.1 Clinical characteristics of the most frequently encountered orofacial pain conditions

Orofacial pain condition	Pain quality	Pain location	Timing/pattern	Treatment
Myofascial pain	Deep ache, can be sharp	Along and behind the jaw Other areas can be affected Secondary headaches common Unilateral or bilateral	Often painful in the morning Generally gets worse throughout the day Pain with chewing and talking	Systemic and topical antiinflammatory therapy Splint therapy Soft diet Physical therapy Other pharmacologic agents (e.g., anxiolytics, muscle relaxants)
Temporo-mandibular joint pain	Sharp	In TMJ Often radiates to the ear Unilateral or bilateral	Worse with opening/closing	Systemic, topical, and intracapsular antiinflammatory therapy Moist heat Soft diet
Atypical facial pain	Dull ache, crushing, burning	Poorly localized Often in the area of a tooth, extracted tooth, or previous surgical procedure Unilateral more common, but can cross midline	Continuous or intermittent throughout the day	Tricyclic antidepressants Second-line agents (clonazepam, gabapentin) Topical compounded agents
Burning mouth syndrome	Burning Sensations of "coated" and "dry" also common Bitter or metallic taste common	Tongue Inner lips Anterior hard palate Throat can be involved Bilateral most common	Continuous, or progressive throughout the day Can have symptom-free days	Clonazepam (systemic and topical)
Trigeminal neuralgia	Sharp, electric shock-like	May begin localized but spreads rapidly Unilateral	Unpredictable May be triggered by light touch or movement Lasts seconds	Anticonvulsants
Odontologic pain	Ranges from dull ache to sharp and pounding	In location of tooth Unilateral	Stimulated by hot/cold Can be spontaneous	Definitive dental therapy

other sites of pain; previous pain history; social history (including major life events); and sleep history. Psychiatric history is also important; specifically regarding treatment for anxiety, depression, and panic attacks, all of which can be associated with chronic pain conditions. A pain score using a 0–10 numerical scale with descriptors should be obtained consistently at each visit (Fig. 10.1).

A careful history accompanied by a comprehensive examination in most cases is sufficient to determine the correct diagnosis, although laboratory tests and imaging studies may be indicated on occasion. Careful explanation of the diagnosis and establishment of real-istic treatment goals are critically important. For example, with neuropathic pain conditions, 50% improvement in symptoms would be considered a very good response; even this may take several trials of medications in different combinations to achieve. All patients should be counseled on responsible use and storage of prescription medications. Nonpharmacologic methods of coping with pain should also be discussed. Patients receiving ongoing treatment should be monitored closely to provide the greatest chance of successful outcome. Use of an accepted metric, such as the above-mentioned pain scale, is necessary to objectively assess the result of treatment.

Fig. 10.1 Pain scale numbered from 0 to 10 with corresponding face pictures and descriptors.

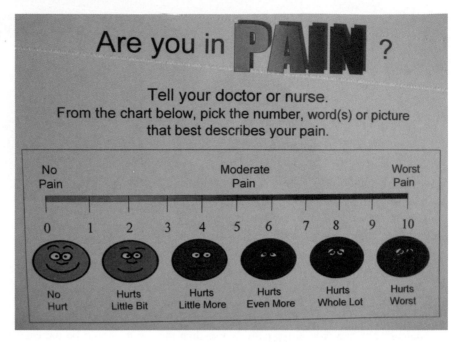

10.2 Odontogenic Pain

As dental infections are common, these must always be included in the differential diagnosis for orofacial pain (see Chap. 7). Pain due to dental caries is quite variable, and depends on such factors as the proximity of decay to the dental pulp, pulp vitality, and presence of a periapical abscess. Hot or cold sensitivity that quickly resolves when the stimulus is removed is characteristic of reversible pulpal inflammation. Spontaneous, pounding pain often occurs once the pulp has become severely inflamed or necrotic. Formation of a periapical abscess may cause pain with chewing and when the tooth is *percussed* (tapped gently with a dental instrument). Although uncommon, *referred pain* to an adjacent tooth or even a tooth in the opposing arch can occur.

In contrast, pain secondary to periodontal disease is typically dull, generalized to a larger area, and more constant. Some patients may complain of generalized cold sensitivity, which is due to loss of periodontal ligament attachment and exposure of the sensitive root surface. Periodontal abscesses can be sharply painful. Odontogenic pain unrelated to infection can be caused by a small crack in a tooth or maladjustment of the occlusion. If there is any concern regarding an odontogenic etiology, patients should be referred to a dentist for evaluation.

Diagnostic tests: Comprehensive dental evaluation including visual inspection, percussion, palpation, pulp vitality testing, periodontal probing, and dental radiographs.
Biopsy: No.
Treatment: Definitive treatment determined by specific diagnosis; see Chap. 7.
Follow-up: Varies with specific nature of problem.

10.3 Myofascial and Temporomandibular Joint Pain

The myofascial and temporomandibular joint (TMJ) and muscles of mastication function together as a unit that is one of the most heavily utilized structures in the human body. Overuse in the form of *parafunctional* activities, which include clenching, bruxism (grinding), and gum chewing is common. Inflammation causes a range of symptoms ranging from mild discomfort to severe debilitating pain. Pain can arise from any component of the masticatory system, including bony structures, the fibrous articular disc, ligamentous joint capsule, or muscles and associated fascia; however, the most common presentation is related to the muscles and fascia (*myofascial pain*) with or without associated *joint arthralgia*. History and careful examination are necessary to determine the correct diagnosis and provide appropriate therapy. In most cases, conservative nonsurgical measures are effective.

10.3.1   History and Examination

In addition to the required elements of a pain history described earlier, patients should be asked specifically if the pain is worse in the morning (typical of nocturnal bruxism), with chewing, or specifically with the act of opening and/or closing the mouth. A history of previous similar episodes, even if less severe, is also important.

Pain is typically described as dull and aching, and radiation throughout the entire side of the face including the temporal region and neck may occur. Pain can be bilateral, but one side is typically worse than the other. Many patients are seen initially by an otolaryngologist if referred ear pain is the main presenting symptom. The most common source of pain in the joint area and ear is arthralgia, which may be associated with some degree of disc derangement (see Chap. 1). Pain is often exacerbated with biting, chewing, talking for extended periods of time, or simply opening and closing the mouth. Patients with osteoarthritis and rheumatoid arthritis may experience pain from joint inflammation or actual bony destruction.

Patients should be examined for facial symmetry. Masseteric hypertrophy may be evident and is characterized by visibly enlarged muscles (Fig. 10.2).

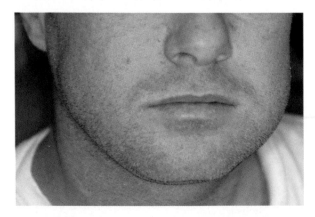

Fig. 10.2 Masseteric hypertrophy in a patient with chronic myofascial pain disorder.

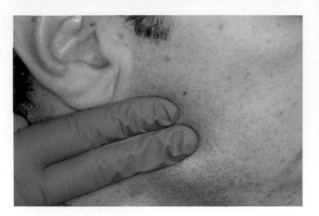

Fig. 10.3 Extraoral palpation of the masseter muscle. Sufficient pressure should be applied to assess for tenderness.

The patient is asked to open and close repeatedly to look for limitation in opening, guarding, or deviation to the right or left. The masseter and all muscles of mastication should be palpated for tenderness (Fig. 10.3; see Chap. 3). The masseter and majority of the temporalis muscle can be palpated extraorally. Intraorally, the medial pterygoid muscle and mandibular attachment of the temporalis can be palpated by inserting the index finger into the posterior maxillary vestibule. Throughout the physical examination, it is important to ask the patient if they note any particular areas of tenderness or sharp pain areas, known as *trigger points*.

The TMJ is palpated initially with the mouth in the closed position (Fig. 10.4). With the first and second fingers positioned over the joint, the patient should then be asked to open and close repeatedly, assessing for pain as well as any symptomatic clicking or *crepitus*.

Trismus, or limited mouth opening, is a potential complication of myofascial and TMJ pain disorders. Trismus can be due to myofascial inflammation with muscle guarding, or less frequently due to a displaced articular disc without *reduction* (see Chap. 1). In the latter case, the disc in the affected joint is unable to translate forward with the mandibular condyle along the articular eminence during mouth opening. The joint on the unaffected side typically opens fully, but deviates painfully to the opposite side. The easiest way to evaluate mouth opening is with a ruler or commercially available triangular measuring device (Fig. 10.5).

Radiographic studies are not routinely obtained in patients presenting with typical signs and symptoms of myofascial and TMJ pain. Plain films have limited

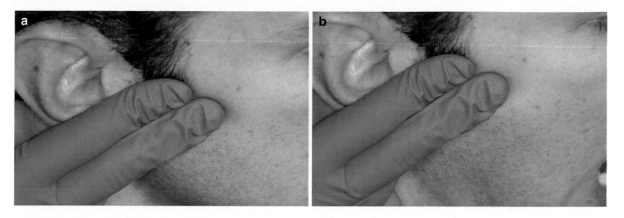

Fig. 10.4 Palpation of the temporomandibular joint (**a**) in the closed position, and (**b**) in the open position. Tenderness in this area generally indicates inflammation of the joint capsule.

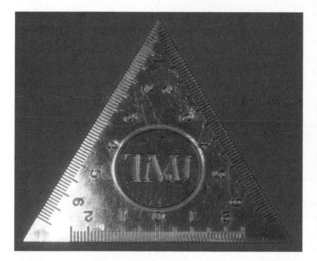

Fig. 10.5 Device used to measure mouth opening. The end of the triangle is inserted between the central incisors and recorded at the maximum interincisal opening in millimeters or centimeters.

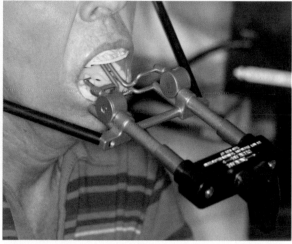

Fig. 10.6 Patient with progressive systemic sclerosis and secondary trismus using a commercially available physical therapy device to increase mouth opening.

benefit in these cases. CT may be useful to assess the degree of joint destruction in patients with arthritic conditions. The use of MRI is reserved for patients with evidence of disc derangement or displacement that fail initial conservative approaches to therapy.

10.3.2   Treatment

The mainstays of treatment include nonsteroidal antiinflammatory agents (NSAIDs) and limitation of nonessential jaw movement. Patients should be instructed to avoid

foods that require forceful biting and chewing, keep their teeth apart except while eating, and minimize parafunctional habits such as gum chewing, clenching, or chewing on other objects. Ice packs may be of some use.

In cases of myofascial pain, physical therapy with passive jaw stretching exercises should also be prescribed, with or without the use of moist heat packs (Fig. 10.6). The jaw is gently and progressively stretched open using the fingers or a prescribed device (Therabite, Atos Medical Inc., West Allis, WI; Dynasplint, Dynasplint Systems, Inc., Severna Park, MD). This is done to the point where it is just uncomfortable and held for 10 seconds with 5–10 repetitions; this sequence is repeated

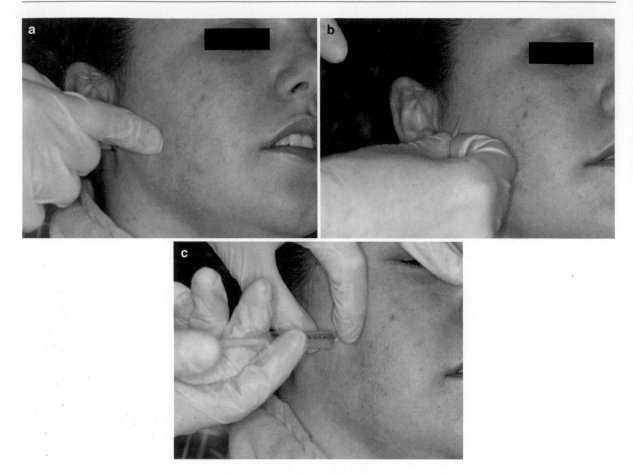

Fig. 10.7 Trigger point injection of the masseter muscle. (**a**) Identification of the trigger point. (**b**) The skin is cleaned with alcohol. (**c**) Injection of combined triamcinolone/mepivacaine directly into the muscle.

several times throughout the day. To avoid systemic complications of long-term NSAID therapy, topical preparations, such as 20% ketoprofen, can be prescribed through a compounding pharmacy and applied several times throughout the day to the affected areas. During acutely painful episodes, a brief course of systemic corticosteroids can be helpful in initially decreasing the inflammation while initiating other measures.

When there is marked arthralgia, or when myofascial trigger points are identified, intralesional corticosteroid therapy can be very effective. The TMJ capsule or trigger point is carefully palpated and injected with 12–16 mg of triamcinolone acetonide (40 mg/mL), using a tuberculin syringe (Fig. 10.7). In some cases, immediate relief is noted. Myofascial trigger points can also be injected with a long-lasting anesthetic such as bupivacaine, either alone or in combination with triam-

cinolone (in a 1:1 ratio). Patients with significant disc derangement and pain whose symptoms do not improve with conservative measures should be referred to an oral and maxillofacial surgeon for evaluation regarding *arthrocentesis* of the TMJ, which is a minimally invasive surgical procedure.

Patients with a history of bruxism may benefit from a custom fabricated occlusal splint, which functions by reducing the overall load on the muscles and TMJ during nocturnal grinding. The splint should provide full occlusal coverage with contact on all teeth to avoid any movement of teeth or adverse affect on the patient's bite, or *occlusion*. The appliance can be designed to fit either the upper or lower teeth. Patients who clench during the day may also benefit from such an appliance, as it can serve as an effective reminder to keep the teeth apart.

Medications directed at reducing parafunctional activity should be considered in some cases. Low dose clonazepam (0.5–1.0 mg) or lorazepam (1.0–2.0 mg) at night before bed can improve sleep, decrease jaw activity, and provide analgesia. Muscle relaxants are similarly used but can be more sedating. In cases of severe pain, short courses of opioid analgesics may be necessary but should not be used for long-term management due to addiction potential.

All patients require careful follow-up, and should be seen regularly until their condition is stable. Any patient on long-term pharmacologic therapy should be evaluated on a regular basis and reassessed for the need for continued therapy.

> **Diagnostic tests**: In most cases none.
> **Biopsy**: No.
> **Treatment**: Must be directed toward the specific diagnosis. Therapies for myofascial pain and arthralgia include systemic and topical NSAID therapy, soft diet, reducing parafunctional activity, splint therapy, passive stretching exercises, anxiolytics and muscle relaxants, systemic and intralesional corticosteroid therapy.
> **Follow-up**: All patients require short- and long-term follow-up.

10.4 Atypical Facial Pain

Atypical facial pain (AFP), sometimes referred to as *persistent idiopathic facial pain* or *atypical odontalgia*, is a neuropathic pain condition that is often mistakenly attributed to dental pathology and can be difficult to diagnose. The pain is typically dull, aching, or burning, and occurs intermittently or constantly throughout the day. The area affected is often poorly defined; over time it can spread or move, in some cases from one side of the face to the other. Intraoral symptoms are often initially associated with a tooth or extraction site, or arise in an area following some type of surgical therapy. Comprehensive dental evaluation is, therefore, a significant component of the work-up of a patient suspected to have AFP. In fact, many patients are treated unnecessarily with root canal (*endodontic*) therapy or extraction of otherwise healthy teeth, after which symptoms persist. There is a strong association with a history of anxiety/depression in patients with AFP.

The pain associated with AFP tends to respond most reliably to low-dose tricyclic antidepressants, including amitryptiline and nortriptyline. If insufficient, addition of either gabapentin or clonazepam generally provides further improvement. Topical medications, including capsaicin and clonazepam, can be prepared by a compounding pharmacist for intra- or extra-oral use. Given the association with a history of anxiety/depression, nonpharmacologic strategies must also be considered.

> **Diagnostic tests**: None specifically. Must obtain appropriate radiographs and perform comprehensive dental evaluation when pain appears to be associated with a tooth.
> **Biopsy**: No.
> **Treatment**: Low dose tricyclic antidepressants, clonazepam, gabapentin. Consider topical compounded formulations.
> **Follow-up**: Patients should be followed carefully until stable response is achieved, then seen at least twice annually.

10.5 Trigeminal Neuralgia

Trigeminal neuralgia is characterized by severe unilateral paroxysmal electric shock-like pain that typically affects one division of the trigeminal nerve. The frequency of attacks is highly variable and symptoms may be quite debilitating. Pain can be stimulated by light touch of the trigger zone or by specific movements, such as smiling or chewing. In most cases, brain MRI is normal; however, vascular compression of the trigeminal ganglion is thought to be the most frequent underlying etiology. Occasionally localized peripheral pathology, such as osteomyelitis or a neoplasm, can result in secondary trigeminal neuralgia (Fig. 10.8). The prevalence of trigeminal neuralgia increases with age. Trigeminal neuralgia can be a feature of multiple sclerosis (although rarely a presenting symptom) and this should be considered in younger patients, particularly females. Clinical variants affecting other cranial nerves include *glossopharyngeal neuralgia* and *occipital neuralgia* also exist.

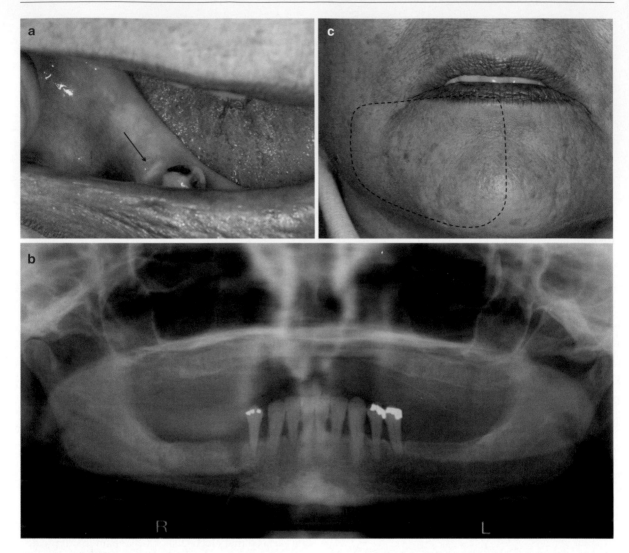

Fig. 10.8 Trigeminal neuralgia secondary to bisphosphonate-associated osteonecrosis of the mandible. (**a**) Area of exposed necrotic bone in the area of the previously extracted second premolar (*arrow*). (**b**) Persistent socket and bone sclerosis involving the area of the right mental formen (*arrow*). (**c**) The anatomic distribution of sharp shooting "electric shock-like" pain in the area innervated by the mental nerve; combined treatment with carbamezapine and gabapentin provided virtually complete resolution of symptoms.

First line therapy for trigeminal neuralgia is carbamazepine, and reduction or elimination of symptoms in response to this medication is diagnostic. The response to anticonvulsants is so predictable that the diagnosis should be reconsidered in those without any evidence of improvement. Other effective medications, typically given in addition to carbamezapine, include gabapentin and baclofen. After several months of sta-bility, the dose and/or frequency of therapy can be carefully reduced; however, it should be increased again if symptoms recur.

Surgical therapies include radiofrequency ablation of the ganglion, nerve blocks, and microvascular decompression. Although these can be effective, patients often have residual symptoms and there is risk of permanent complications.

Diagnostic tests: Consider brain MRI to rule-out neoplasm or systemic disease such as multiple sclerosis, especially in younger individuals.

Biopsy: No.

Treatment: Medical therapies include carbamezapine, gabapentin, and baclofen. Refractory cases should be referred for neurosurgical consultation.

Follow-up: Patients must be followed carefully for response to medical therapy and adjustment of medications as needed. Dosage can be tapered after a stable response has been maintained for at least 3 months.

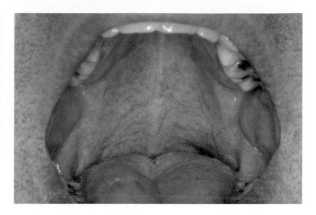

Fig. 10.9 Prominent palatal vasculature interpreted as "lacerations" following oral self-examination by a patient with burning mouth syndrome

10.6 Burning Mouth Syndrome

Burning mouth syndrome (BMS), also referred to as *stomatodynia*, is characterized by burning dysesthesia that most commonly affects the tongue, but can also involve the inner aspect of the lips and anterior hard palate. The majority of patients are peri- and postmenopausal women; however, men and younger patients of both sexes can be affected. Most patients have a significant history of anxiety, depression, or panic attacks, and the onset of symptoms often correlates with a major life event or particularly stressful period in life. It is not uncommon for patients to see multiple providers, have numerous tests performed, receive treatment for various "infections," and ultimately be told that there is "nothing wrong" and no treatment is available. This only further increases their anxiety and emotional distress.

The pain is typically described as a "burning" or "scalded" sensation, but some may describe the tissues as feeling "different," "swollen," "tingling," or "itchy." Pain can be so severe as to be rated greater than 10 out of 10 on a 0–10 scale (where 10 is the worst pain they have ever experienced). It often becomes a fixation that the patient cannot ignore, interfering with daily activities and job responsibilities. Although the pain is almost always spontaneous, certain spicy and acidic foods can exacerbate symptoms. In most patients, however, eating or drinking diminishes or eliminates symptoms. Patients often describe observing "sores" or "lesions" on their tongue; however, these findings are invariably normal components of the tongue anatomy, such as papillae and vessels (Fig. 10.9; see Chap. 1).

Although there are several clinical patterns of BMS, most patients become aware of burning at some point soon after waking up. The pain usually persists throughout the day, generally becoming more severe toward evening. Altered taste, typically described as "bitter" or "metallic," as well as complaint of xerostomia (despite normal objective salivary function), are both common symptoms associated with BMS. Patients may occasionally describe an associated sensation of throat constriction, presence of a "lump" in the throat, or fear that they will not be able to breathe or swallow; clinical examination is invariably normal. Sleeping disturbances are also quite common in patients with BMS, characterized by difficulty falling asleep or waking easily and frequently throughout the night.

The diagnosis of BMS is one of exclusion. Clinical examination is within normal limits. Other causes of oral burning, such as infection, mucosal disease, uncontrolled diabetes, thyroid disease, and hematologic disorders, must be sufficiently ruled out. Precise guidelines for ordering such tests are vague and should be guided by best clinical judgment. It is critical for the medical provider to acknowledge that the pain is real, that the patient is not "making up" the condition, and that BMS is a well-recognized disorder. It is also important to explain that there is no way to predict how long the condition will last, but that therapy is available.

The first line medication for BMS, especially when patients report a significant history of sleep disturbance, is clonazepam, which can be prescribed systemically and/or topically. The starting dose for systemic therapy is typically 0.5 mg just before bed, and most patients tolerate this dose without complication. If necessary, the tablet can be cut in half to reduce the dose to 0.25 mg.

For patients who do not have sleep disturbances or are reluctant to take the medication systemically, topical clonazepam can be very effective. This is administered either by dissolving a tablet in the mouth or rinsing with a specially compounded solution.

All patients should be reevaluated after 1 month of therapy and the regimen adjusted as necessary. Depending on the tolerability of systemic therapy, sleep quality, and breakthrough of symptoms later in the day, the regimen can be altered as follows: the evening systemic dose can be increased (typically from 0.5 to 1.0 mg), a second systemic dose can be added midday (typically 0.5 mg), or topical therapy can be added if not already being used. Patients should be evaluated monthly until a stable response is achieved, then every 6 months.

For those who do not respond, or have an insufficient response with clonazepam, second line agents include gabapentin and the tricyclic antidepressants. Although there are no reports in the literature, it is likely that these agents may also be effective topically. Evidence supporting the use of alpha lipoic acid, an over the counter supplement, is weak. Topical capsaicin applied repeatedly over an extended period of time can effectively deplete substance P production resulting in periods of remission. This is easily prepared at home by mixing 3–4 drops of hot sauce in a teaspoon of water and rinsing for several minutes, 2–3 times a day. Alternatively, a compounding pharmacy can prepare a 0.05% rinse or gel. The effectiveness of complementary and alternative therapies, such as acupuncture and hypnosis, is unclear.

Diagnostic tests: None in most cases.
Biopsy: No.
Treatment: Patient education is critical. First-line therapy with clonazepam (systemic and/or topical); second-therapy with gabapentin and tricyclic antidepressants. Topical capsaicin therapy can be offered; however, long-term compliance is generally poor.
Follow-up: Monthly until a stable response is achieved, then twice yearly.

Sources

Clark GT. Persistent orodental pain, atypical odontalgia, and phantom tooth pain: when are they neuropathic disorders? J Calif Dent Assoc 2006;34:599–609

Lewis MA, Sankar V, De Laat A, Benoliel R. Management of neuropathic orofacial pain. Oral Surg Oral Med Oral Pathol Oral Radiol Endod 2007;103 Suppl:S32.e1–24

Maltsman-Tseikhin A, Moricca P, Niv D. Burning mouth syndrome: will better understanding yield better management? Pain Pract 2007;7(2):151–62

Matwychuk MJ. Diagnostic challenges of neuropathic tooth pain. J Can Dent Assoc 2004;70:542–6

Okeson JP. Orofacial Pain: Guidelines for Assessment, Diagnosis, and Management. Quintessence, Carol Stream, IL, 1996

Patton LL, Siegel MA, Benoliel R, De Laat A. Management of burning mouth syndrome: systematic review and management recommendations. Oral Surg Oral Med Oral Pathol Oral Radiol Endod 2007;103 Suppl:S39.e1–13

Scrivani SJ, Keith DA, Kaban LB. Temporomandibular disorders. N Engl J Med 2008;359:2693–705

Siccoli MM, Bassetti CL, Sandor PS. Facial pain: clinical differential diagnosis. Lancet Neurol 2006;5:257–67

Chapter 11
Oral Manifestations of Systemic Disease

Summary Lesions inside the oral cavity can be associated with a number of systemic conditions, representing important indicators of active disease or heralding the onset of disease. Recognition of such lesions may facilitate prompt diagnosis and treatment of underlying disease with overall improvement in patients' quality of life. In some cases, oral findings persist despite adequate systemic management of disease, necessitating targeted ancillary care measures. This chapter reviews the presentation and management of oral findings that may be seen in association with systemic conditions, including autoimmune, gastrointestinal, and granulomatous disorders.

Keywords Systemic lupus erythematosus • Lichenoid inflammation • Sjögren syndrome • Discoid lupus • Scleroderma • Graft-versus-host disease • Inflammatory bowel disease • Crohn disease • Angular cheilitis • Orofacial granulomatosis • Ulcerative colitis • Pyostomatitis vegetans • Gardner syndrome • Peutz-Jeghers syndrome • Wegener granulomatosis • Antineutrophilic cytoplasmic antibody • Sarcoidosis • Heerfordt syndrome • Angiotensin converting enzyme • Human immunodeficiency syndrome • Iron deficiency anemia • Plummer-Vinson syndrome • Pernicious anemia • Intrinsic factor • Thrombocytopenia • Cyclic neutropenia • Lymphoma • Midline lethal granuloma • Leukemia • Cowden syndrome • Jaundice • Bisphosphonate-associated osteonecrosis • Sequestra

11.1   Introduction

Lesions inside the oral cavity can be associated with a number of systemic conditions, representing important indicators of active disease or heralding the onset of disease. Recognition of such lesions may facilitate prompt diagnosis and treatment of underlying disease with overall improvement in patient quality of life. In some cases, oral findings persist despite adequate systemic management of disease, necessitating targeted ancillary care measures. Management of these patients typically requires careful and close collaboration with other medical specialists for appropriate coordination of care and follow-up.

11.2   Autoimmune Diseases

11.2.1   Systemic Lupus Erythematosus

Production of autoantibodies to nuclear proteins in systemic lupus erythematosus (SLE) results in a chronic inflammatory condition with immune complex deposition that can affect any tissue in the body. Symptoms vary widely, and the disease may follow an unpredictable course with relapses and remissions over a long period of time. Organs most commonly involved include the heart, skin, joints, kidney, and nervous system. Young women are most often affected, with peak age of onset between 15 and 40 years of age. An erythematous malar "butterfly" rash (Fig. 11.1) may be seen across the nose and cheeks in 30–60% of patients, which can intensify with sun exposure. The mainstays of treatment include high-dose steroids and other immunosuppressive and immunomodulatory agents.

Oral findings occur in up to 40% of patients with SLE, and their presence can be important in helping to initially establish the diagnosis. The appearance of

J.M. Bruch and N.S. Treister, *Clinical Oral Medicine and Pathology,*
DOI 10.1007/978-1-60327-520-0_11, © Humana Press, a part of Springer Science+Business Media, LLC 2010

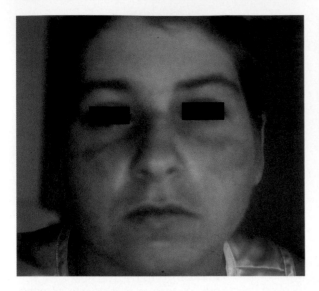

Fig. 11.1 Typical "butterfly" rash in a patient with systemic lupus erythematosus. Photograph courtesy of Stephen Sonis, DMD, DMSc, Boston, MA.

Diagnostic Tests: Medical work-up for SLE including measurement of antibodies (such as antinuclear antibody, antidouble-stranded DNA, lupus anticoagulant, anticardiolipin antibody) and complement.

Biopsy: Can be helpful in establishing a diagnosis. Immunofluorescence ("lupus band test") shows linear band-like deposition of immunoreactants along basement membrane.

Treatment: Avoidance of sun exposure. Use of systemic steroidal and nonsteroidal antiinflammatory agents, topical steroids, anti-malarials (hydroxychloroquine) for minor inflammatory or non major organ involvement. Use of high-dose systemic steroids (prednisone) and cytotoxic/immunosuppressive medications (cyclophosphamide, azathioprine, mycophenolate mofetil) for major organ system involvement.

Follow-up: Close follow-up to monitor activity of disease and medications.

oral lesions varies, without any one defining or common feature. *Lichenoid inflammation*, presenting with areas of erythema, ulceration, and white striations are most common (Fig. 11.2). *Aphthous-like* ulcerations or *granulomatous swellings* may also be seen. *Sjögren syndrome* is common in patients with SLE and can develop at any point during the course of the disease (see Chap. 8). Hematologic abnormalities are frequently present in patients with active SLE, and oral hematomas may be observed in thrombocytopenic patients (Fig. 11.3).

11.2.2 Chronic Cutaneous Lupus Erythematosus

This is also known as *Discoid lupus* and affects the skin without visceral involvement; however, it can progress to SLE in a minority of patients. Thick scaly red patches occur on the scalp and face, which may scar or result in areas of hypopigmentation. Oral lesions can be seen on the buccal mucosa appearing as erythematous plaques with white striations that look

Fig. 11.2 Lichenoid appearing ulcerations of the ventral tongue in a patient with systemic lupus erythematosus. Photograph courtesy of Stephen Sonis, DMD, DMSc, Boston, MA.

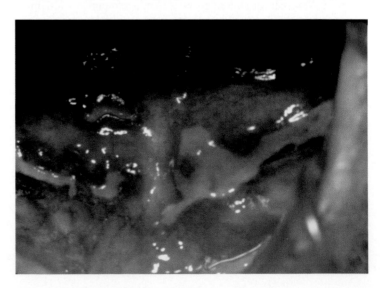

Fig. 11.3 Hematomas of the labial mucosa in a patient with thrombocytopenia secondary to a flare of her systemic lupus erythematosus.

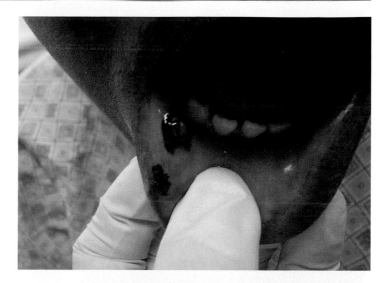

clinically identical to oral lichen planus (see Chap. 5); ulceration may also be present.

> **Diagnostic Tests**: Generally no serologic findings as would be seen with SLE. Diagnosis is often based on the clinical appearance of skin lesions.
> **Biopsy**: As above with SLE.
> **Treatment**: Avoid exposure to Sun. Use of topical agents; systemic medications if refractory.
> **Follow-up**: Monitor activity of disease and response to medications.

11.2.3 Progressive Systemic Sclerosis

Progressive systemic sclerosis, or *scleroderma*, is a rare autoimmune disease with the main feature consisting of progressive fibrosis of the skin and connective tissue resulting in significant disfigurement and disability. Other affected organs include the lungs, kidneys, heart, digestive system, muscles, and nervous system. Patients often develop restricted mouth opening secondary to fibrosis of the facial skin and perioral tissues, making eating, speaking, and maintenance of oral hygiene extremely challenging (Figs. 11.4 and 11.5). Associated myofascial and temporomandibular joint pain is common. Dysphagia is also a frequent complication due to fibrosis and constriction of the esophagus as well as decreased salivary flow secondary to possible associated Sjögren syndrome. Management of oral complications includes

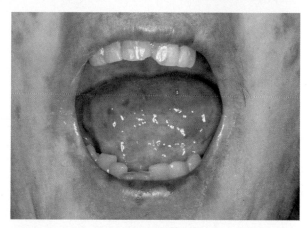

Fig. 11.4 Limited mouth opening due to fibrosis and contracture of the perioral soft tissue in a patient with progressive systemic sclerosis.

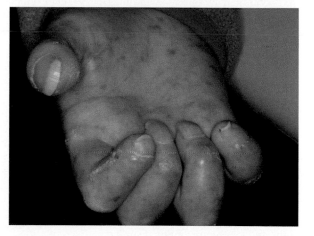

Fig. 11.5 Contracture and deformity of the hands in a patient with progressive systemic sclerosis making a simple daily activity such as brushing the teeth severely challenging.

jaw stretching exercises (see Fig. 10.6), treatment of xerostomia-related symptoms, use of an electric toothbrush, and frequent dental visits. Unfortunately, there is no treatment; management is palliative.

Diagnostic Tests: Rheumatologic evaluation, including serologic testing (ESR, RF, ANA, anti-centromere antibody, SCL-70/scleroderma antibody). Evaluation of organ systems as indicated: pulmonary function testing, CXR, barium swallow, etc.

Biopsy: Skin biopsy will show characteristic fibrotic changes; however, this is generally not needed for diagnosis.

Treatment: None specifically; Symptomatic treatment of complications (dysphagia, pulmonary hypertension, Raynaud's, etc.). Use of immunomodulatory (prednisone, methotrexate, chlorambucil, cyclosporine, tacrolimus) or antifibrotic (penicillamine, colchicines) agents. See Chapter 10 for trismus management guidelines.

Follow-up: Routine monitoring of disease progression.

11.2.4 Chronic Graft-Versus-Host Disease

Although not a true autoimmune disorder, chronic graft-versus-host disease (cGVHD) is in many ways quite similar. Allogeneic hematopoietic cell transplantation is utilized to treat a number of hematologic malignancies and bone marrow failure syndromes. cGVHD develops in greater than 50% of these patients, usually within 6–12 months of transplantation, and frequently involves the oral cavity, skin, liver, and eyes. Alloreactive donor T cells recognize host tissue antigens as "foreign" and mount an immune response to the host tissue that mimics a variety of autoimmune diseases. In addition to systemic immunomodulatory therapy, many patients require intensive organ specific ancillary treatment for management of their symptoms. Although allogeneic hematopoietic cell transplantation is only performed in highly specialized medical centers, most patients return to their local communities for follow-up care, so it is essential that their doctors are able to recognize the signs and symptoms of this disorder.

Oral cGVHD targets the mucosa and salivary glands. In some cases, these may be the initial (or only) sites exhibiting findings. Mucosal lesions are essentially identical to those of *oral lichen planus* (see Chap. 5) and are characterized clinically by reticulation, erythema, and ulceration (Fig. 11.6). *Superficial mucoceles* (see Chap. 8) of the palate, or less frequently on the labial and buccal mucosa, are common and are caused by inflammation of the minor salivary glands (Fig. 11.7). These noninfectious submucosal vesicles often develop acutely during meals, are generally more annoying than painful, and resolve spontaneously within hours to days. If the major salivary glands are involved, patients may complain of xerostomia; the presentation in these cases is similar to that seen with *Sjögren syndrome* and patients are at significantly increased risk for developing rampant dental caries (Fig. 11.8). Diagnosis of oral cGVHD is primarily based on history and clinical examination.

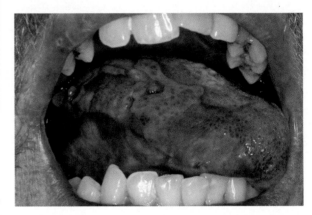

Fig. 11.6 Large ulceration with erythema and reticulation of the tongue in a patient with severe oral chronic graft-versus-host disease.

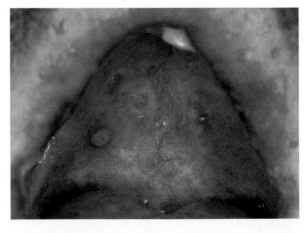

Fig. 11.7 Multiple superficial mucoceles of the palate with associated reticulation in a patient with chronic graft-versus-host disease.

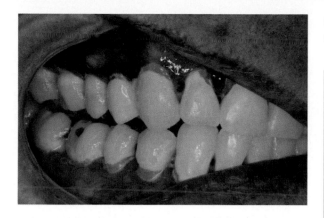

Fig. 11.8 Extensive cervical decay in a patient with oral chronic graft-versus-host disease. The dental decay developed less than 2 years following transplantation, prior to which there was no evidence of caries.

Treatment of mucosal lesions includes use of topical steroids and topical tacrolimus, both of which are easily and effectively applied in rinse form, especially when disease is extensive. Tacrolimus ointment works well for lesions on the lips. Salivary gland disease can be managed with prescription sialogogue therapy as well as over the counter dry mouth treatments. Patients with any evidence of salivary gland disease should receive daily topical fluoride therapy. Dental caries should be treated aggressively, and dental radiographs should be obtained annually to monitor for new carious lesions.

Patients with a history of allogeneic hematopoietic cell transplantation and cGVHD have a significantly increased risk for developing oral *squamous cell carcinoma* (see Chap. 9). Even if asymptomatic, all patients must receive an annual oral cancer screening and any suspicious lesions should be biopsied (Fig. 11.9).

Diagnostic tests: None. Consider viral culture of ulcerative lesions to rule out HSV infection.

Biopsy: No, unless diagnosis of cGVHD is unclear or there is concern for malignancy.

Treatment: Treatment is directed at managing symptoms. Many patients require intensive local therapy in addition to systemic immunosuppressive treatment.

For *mucosal disease*: Topical dexamethasone and tacrolimus rinses, which can be used in combination (swish for 5 min then spit, up to six times daily). Painful ulcerative lesions may benefit from intralesional triamcinolone therapy as well as intensive topical therapy with clobetasol gel. Use of mild toothpaste is effective for patients with toothpaste sensitivity. Depending on symptoms, patients should be advised to avoid acidic, spicy, and hard or crusty foods as well as carbonated beverages.

For *salivary gland disease*: Over the counter lubricant rinses and gels as well as use of sugar-free gum and candy can be helpful. Prescription sialogogue therapy with cevimeline or pilocarpine is available. All patients should receive daily prescription topical fluoride (5,000 ppm). Regular dental visits with radiographic evaluation are necessary to identify and treat xerostomia-related dental caries.

Follow-up: Initially close follow-up to assess response to therapy, then annually for oral cancer screening and dental exam.

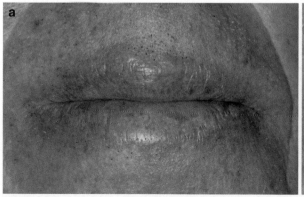

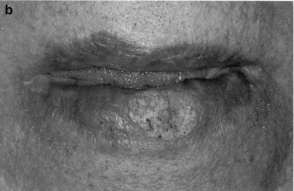

Fig. 11.9 Risk of malignant transformation in chronic graft-versus-host disease. (**a**) Prominent reticulation of the lips that was symptomatic and responded well to topical tacrolimus therapy. (**b**) Development of a large, focal, verrucous leukoplakia 7 months later that demonstrated dysplasia histopathologically. This was treated with wide excision followed by topical therapy with 5-fluorouracil.

11.3 Gastrointestinal Disorders

Oral lesions may be seen with a variety of gastrointestinal conditions and often correspond to active disease in the GI tract; however, they can appear prior to other GI manifestations.

11.3.1 *Inflammatory Bowel Disease*

Inflammatory bowel disease refers to a group of disorders causing chronic recurrent ulcerative inflammatory lesions in the gastrointestinal tract, with symptoms that include abdominal cramping, bloating, pain, diarrhea, weight loss, and bleeding.

11.3.1.1 Crohn Disease

This is a granulomatous inflammatory disorder of unknown etiology affecting primarily the distal small intestine, rectum, and proximal colon. Oral lesions may precede onset of GI symptoms or correlate with their activity, underscoring the importance of a good history. *Angular cheilitis* (see Chap. 7) may be evident, likely secondary to a combination of immunosuppressive therapy and malabsorption. Extension of mucosal inflammation to the oral cavity can result in edema or ulceration of the lips (Fig. 11.10). These lesions are virtually identical to those seen in idiopathic *orofacial granulomatosis* (see later and Chap. 5). Intraorally, the gingiva and buccal mucosa may exhibit hyperplasia and fissuring, with a thickened or "cobblestoned" appearance (Fig. 11.11). Aphthous-like ulcers may be present, which can be severe (Figs. 11.12 and 11.13).

Oral lesions can be treated with topical or systemic steroids. Management of intestinal symptoms involves the use of systemic medications including steroids, sulfasalazine, immunosuppressant agents, and anti-TNF-alpha biological agents. Surgical resection of portions of the bowel or rectum is necessary in some cases; however, concurrent oral manifestations may not improve following such intervention.

Diagnostic Tests: Medical work-up with endoscopy and radiographic testing as indicated.

Biopsy: Histology is nonspecific, showing non-necrotizing granulomatous inflammation. Biopsy of oral lesions may support the diagnosis in conjunction with history and GI findings or suggest the diagnosis in absence of GI signs or symptoms.

Treatment: Topical steroids for oral lesions (see guidelines in Chap. 5 for recurrent aphthous stomatitis and orofacial granulomatosis); systemic steroids or azathioprine if refractory. For angular cheilitis, see guidelines in Chap. 7.

Follow-up: Regular follow-up to monitor activity of disease and tolerance of medications.

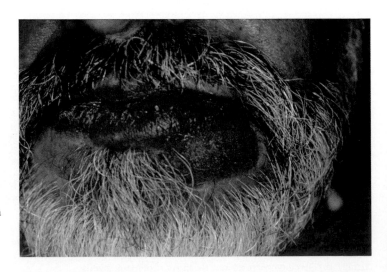

Fig. 11.10 Granulomatous inflammation of the lips and perioral skin with swelling and erythema in a patient with Crohn disease. Photograph courtesy of Sook-Bin Woo, DMD, MMSc, Boston, MA.

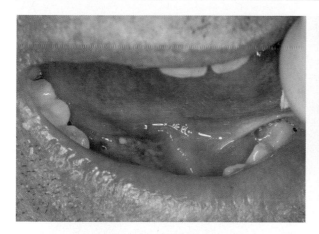

Fig. 11.11 Deeply fissured aphthous-like ulceration in a patient with otherwise well-controlled Crohn disease.

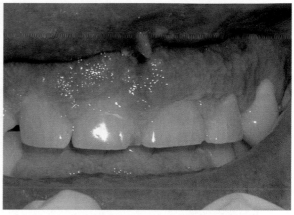

Fig. 11.14 Pyostomatitis vegetans in a patient with ulcerative colitis demonstrating multiple yellowish white pustules on the labial and alveolar mucosa. Photograph courtesy of Scott S. De Rossi, DMD, Augusta, GA.

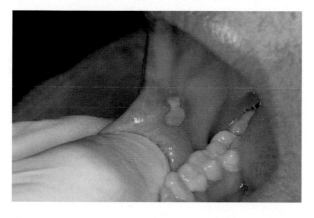

Fig. 11.12 Aphthous-like ulceration in a patient with Crohn disease.

11.3.1.2 Ulcerative Colitis

This condition mainly affects the colon and rectum, with resulting hemorrhagic ulceration of the intestinal lining and abscess formation causing bloody diarrhea, weight loss, and fatigue. Oral manifestations include aphthous-like ulcers, which may coincide with flare-up of GI symptoms. Rarely, multiple small mucosal pustular-appearing lesions resembling "snail tracks" called *pyostomatitis vegetans* may be observed on the palate or buccal mucosa (Fig. 11.14). The treatment for ulcerative colitis involves the use of both topical and systemic steroids.

> **Diagnostic Tests**: As above for Crohn disease. Stool evaluation to rule out infectious causes.
> **Biopsy**: As indicated.
> **Treatment**: As above for Crohn disease.
> **Follow-up**: Monitor activity of disease and medications. Close follow-up secondary to increased risk of colon cancer.

11.3.2 Gardner Syndrome

This is an inherited, autosomal dominant condition characterized by multiple adenomatous colorectal polyps as well as cutaneous cysts and fibromas. The intestinal

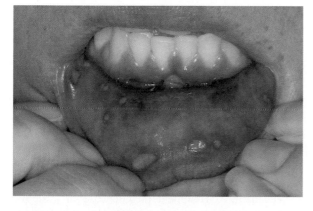

Fig. 11.13 Severe aphthous-ulcerations, some with fissures, in a patient experiencing a flare of Crohn disease.

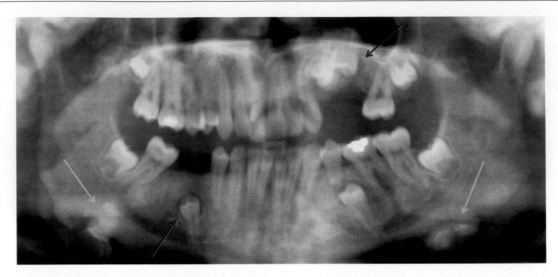

Fig. 11.15 Panoramic radiograph of a patient with Gardner syndrome showing multiple impacted teeth (*red arrows*) and osteomas (*yellow arrows*). Radiograph courtesy of Michael Pharoah, DDS, MSC, Toronto, ON.

lesions demonstrate a very high rate of malignant transformation, and patients will often undergo prophylactic colectomy. Oral manifestations include multiple osteomas of the jaws and facial bones, supernumerary (extra) teeth, impacted teeth, and odontomas (Fig. 11.15). The oral lesions do not have malignant potential.

> **Diagnostic Tests**: GI workup with colonoscopy.
> **Biopsy**: Biopsy of GI lesions.
> **Treatment**: Colectomy due to high risk of malignant transformation. Treatment of extracolonic lesions is necessary only for symptomatic or cosmetic reasons.
> **Follow-up**: Close follow-up of GI lesions secondary to cancer risk.

11.3.3   Peutz-Jeghers Syndrome

This syndrome is characterized by autosomal dominant inheritance, benign intestinal polyps, and pigmented mucosal and cutaneous lesions. Patients are prone to bowel intussusception and are at risk for breast and ovarian cancer. Skin lesions typically present as freckling in the perioral region and may fade with age. Diffuse brown patches can be seen intraorally and may resemble physiologic pigmentation.

> **Diagnostic Tests**: GI workup as indicated.
> **Biopsy**: Oral and skin lesions are benign. Biopsy as indicated of GI or other lesions.
> **Treatment**: Treatment of GI complications and other nonoral manifestations as indicated.
> **Follow-up**: Monitoring for intussusception and tumor formation.

11.4   Granulomatous Diseases

11.4.1   Wegener Granulomatosis

This is an idiopathic, multiorgan system, small vessel granulomatous vasculitis, which mainly affects the upper and lower respiratory tracts and kidneys. Measurement of antineutrophilic cytoplasmic antibody (ANCA) is frequently positive. Oral lesions are not as common as sinonasal manifestations and are very rarely the initial presenting feature of the disease. The most common oral manifestations include mucosal ulcers of the palate or diffuse hyperplastic gingivitis (Fig. 11.16). The latter is sometimes referred to as "strawberry gingivitis" based on the color and pebbly surface texture. Treatment includes use of systemic steroids as well as other immunosuppressive or cytotoxic drugs such as methotrexate and cyclophosph-

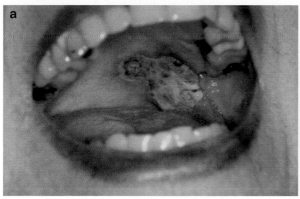
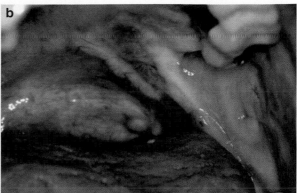

Fig. 11.16 Wegener disease of the palate. (**a**) Necrotic ulceration of the left soft palate diagnosed by histopathology and serology. The patient also had ulcerative lesions of the left tongue and posterior mandibular gingiva. (**b**) Healing lesion 2 months later following high-dose prednisone therapy. Photographs courtesy of Sook-Bin Woo, DMD, MMSc, Boston, MA.

amide. Oral lesions generally improve with treatment of the disease.

> **Diagnostic Tests**: Labwork to evaluate kidney function; c-ANCA; ESR; chest XR; ± sinus films.
> **Biopsy**: Yes; histology shows features of necrotizing granulomatous vasculitis.
> **Treatment**: Systemic medication (steroids, cyclophosphamide, methotrexate). Topical palliative rinses for painful oral lesions.
> **Follow-up**: Close follow-up to monitor activity of disease and medication side effects.

11.4.2 Sarcoidosis

The etiology of this disease is unknown; however, it may represent an immune response to environmental exposures with underlying genetic predisposition. It is characterized by noncaseating granulomas primarily involving pulmonary and lymphoid tissue. However, manifestations can be quite diverse, with involvement of multiple organ systems. It is usually seen in adults under the age of 40, with a higher incidence in females and African Americans. Painless enlargement of salivary tissue, most often the parotid glands, can occur. The triad of parotid involvement, facial nerve weakness, and uveitis is known as *Heerfordt syndrome,* or *uveo-parotid fever.* Oral lesions are rare and can be seen in any location as asymptomatic submucosal masses. Diagnosis is based on clinical findings in conjunction with tissue biopsy.

Levels of angiotensin converting enzyme (ACE) may be elevated in 60–75% of patients; however, this is not pathognomonic for the disease. Depending on severity of symptoms, treatment may involve use of systemic steroids or other immunosuppressive medications.

> **Diagnostic Tests**: Blood tests including ACE, ESR, CBC; chest XR.
> **Biopsy**: Yes; histology shows noncaseating granulomatous inflammation.
> **Treatment**: Mild cases may not require treatment and may resolve spontaneously. Systemic steroids are given for more severe cases; other immunosuppressive medications such as azathioprine, methotrexate, or cyclophosphamide if refractory.
> **Follow-up**: Close follow-up to monitor disease progression and medication side effects.

11.4.3 Orofacial Granulomatosis

This is an inflammatory condition characterized by noncaseating granulomas and nontender swelling of oral and facial soft tissues, most commonly involving the lips. Diagnosis is based on exclusion of other granulomatous inflammatory diseases, such as sarcoid, *Crohn disease*, allergy or foreign body reaction, and mycobacterial infection. This condition as well as its management is discussed in greater detail in Chap. 5.

11.5 Human Immunodeficiency Virus

Treatment with highly active antiretroviral therapy (HAART) has changed the management and prognosis of human immunodeficiency virus (HIV)/AIDS dramatically in recent years. It has also decreased the prevalence of many oral findings associated with this disease in developed countries. HIV infected patients are subject to a variety of opportunistic infections because of diminished cellular immune activity, leading to oral manifestations such as candidiasis and reactivation of HSV and CMV ulcerations (see Chap. 7). Despite advances in management, oral candidiasis is seen commonly in HIV positive patients, and can progress to invasive esophageal candidiasis if not appropriately treated.

Other virally mediated disorders, such as oral hairy leukoplakia related to EBV and Kaposi sarcoma associated with HHV-8, have been discussed elsewhere in the book (see Chaps. 4 and 6). Oral HPV-related lesions, including squamous papillomas and condylomas (see Chap. 7), are found commonly in HIV-positive patients and involvement of the lips and mucosa can be quite extensive (Fig. 11.17).

HIV-positive patients may experience severe necrotizing gingivitis or periodontitis with need for extensive treatment including surgical debridement. They should be followed closely, with meticulous attention to oral hygiene and regular dental care (Fig. 11.18). AIDS patients are also prone to developing large, painful, major aphthous ulcers often requiring treatment with intralesional, topical, and/or systemic corticosteroids (Fig. 11.19). In refractory cases thalidomide, which is FDA approved for this use, should be considered. Of note, the apparent severity of these lesions may parallel worsening immunosuppression.

As with other immunosuppressed individuals, AIDS patients are at increased risk for malignancy, including lymphoma, which is primarily of the non-Hodgkin B cell type. Oral lymphomas may be seen as firm masses or shallow ulcerations anywhere in the oral cavity, although they occur most often on the palate or gingiva (Fig. 11.20). These can present as isolated lesions without disseminated disease or associated constitutional symptoms.

Salivary gland involvement, including unilateral or bilateral parotid enlargement, xerostomia, and benign lymphoepithelial cysts, can be seen. As mentioned previously, xerostomia can result in significant morbidity from dental caries.

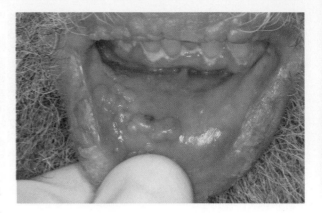
Fig. 11.17 Multiple condylomas of the lower labial mucosa in an HIV positive patient.

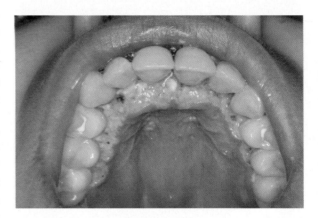
Fig. 11.18 Recrudescent herpes simplex virus infection along the entire gingival margin of the palate following deep dental scaling in a patient with AIDS.

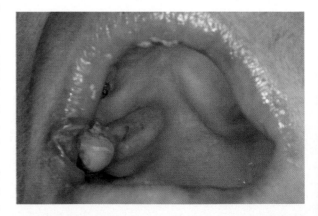
Fig. 11.19 HIV associated major aphthous ulcers of the palate and lip in a patient with advanced AIDS.

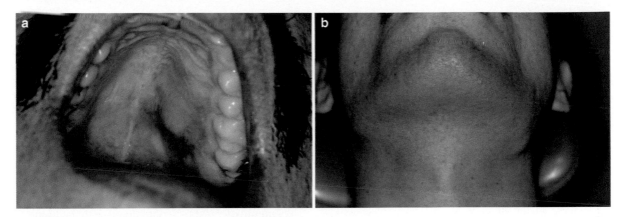

Fig. 11.20 Swelling of the left posterior hard palate (**a**) and left submandibular lymphadenopathy, (**b**) diagnosed histopathologically as non-Hodgkin lymphoma in an HIV positive patient. Photograph courtesy of Sook-Bin Woo, DMD, MMSc, Boston, MA

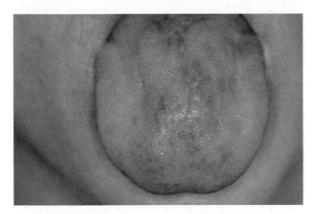

Fig. 11.21 Atrophic glossitis with depapillation and erythema in a patient with iron deficiency anemia.

11.6 Hematologic Disorders

11.6.1 *Anemia*

11.6.1.1 Iron Deficiency Anemia

Iron deficiency, most commonly secondary to either physiologic blood loss in women during menses or pathologic blood loss from the gastrointestinal tract, results in microcytic hypochromic anemia with low serum iron and elevated total iron-binding capacity. Characteristic oral findings include pallor of the lips and mucosa and atrophy of the lingual papillae, with a shiny, "bald" appearance to the tongue dorsum (Fig. 11.21); patients may complain of a burning sensation of the tongue. Iron deficiency anemia is also implicated in a small subset of

patients with recurrent aphthous stomatitis (see Chap. 5).

Chronic severe iron deficiency anemia is seen in *Plummer-Vinson syndrome*, which is associated with dysphagia secondary to esophageal webs and strictures as well as increased risk for squamous cell carcinoma (see Chap. 9) of the upper aerodigestive tract. Oral mucosal atrophy and pain can be quite pronounced. This condition is seen more frequently in women.

> **Diagnostic Tests**: Medical work-up for anemia, fatigue, and occult blood loss.
> **Biopsy**: No.
> **Treatment**: Iron supplementation.
> **Follow-up**: As needed depending on etiology and response to treatment.

11.6.1.2 Pernicious Anemia

Deficiency of *intrinsic factor*, which is produced by parietal cells in the gastric mucosa, results in inability to absorb vitamin B12 from the intestinal mucosa and subsequent vitamin B12 deficiency. The resulting megaloblastic anemia shows a macrocytic, hyperchromic pattern, with decreased serum B12 levels. The tongue dorsum exhibits atrophy of the papillae, with a smooth surface that may be beefy or fiery red and sore. Vitamin B12 deficiency is also associated with a small subset of patients suffering from recurrent aphthous stomatitis.

page 150 Clinical Oral Medicine and Pathology

Diagnostic Tests: Medical work-up for anemia and associated symptoms.
Biopsy: No.
Treatment: B12 supplementation; generally parenteral via injection on a monthly basis.
Follow-up: Regular to monitor treatment.

11.6.2 Thrombocytopenia

A decrease in the number of circulating platelets can result in inadequate hemostasis secondary to impaired clot formation. Small, pinpoint hemorrhagic lesions (*petechiae*) and larger areas of bruising (*ecchymosis*) may be seen in the oral cavity, particularly in areas exposed to masticatory stress such as the tongue, buccal mucosa, and palate (see Chap. 6). Mass-like collections of extravasated blood (*hematomas*) can develop; these range in color from blue, grey, to black, and are characterized by a firm, rubbery consistency (Fig. 11.22). These lesions will not blanch with applied pressure, differentiating them from vascular lesions in which the blood is contained within the vessels, such as hemangiomas (see Chap. 6).

Diagnostic Tests: Laboratory testing to evaluate for underlying bleeding disorder.
Biopsy: No.
Treatment: Management of underlying medical issue, if applicable.
Follow-up: As indicated for specific etiology.

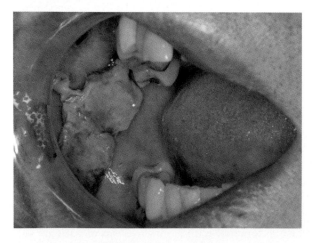

Fig. 11.22 Large hematoma of the right buccal mucosa in a patient with thrombocytopenia.

11.6.3 Cyclic Neutropenia

This is a rare inherited condition in which the circulating neutrophil count fluctuates in a cyclical fashion with a decrease occurring every 21 days and lasting for 3–5 days. Patients are susceptible to infections while the white blood cell count remains low and may report a history of recurrent fever, lymph node enlargement, malaise, and pharyngitis. Oral findings consist mainly of mucosal aphthous-like ulcers, gingivitis, and periodontal disease.

Diagnostic tests: Serial blood testing demonstrating periodic fluctuation of neutrophil levels.
Biopsy: No.
Treatment: Supportive treatment of symptoms. Antibiotics as needed for infection. Consideration for granulocyte colony-stimulating factor (G-CSF).
Follow-up: As needed.

11.7 Malignancy

11.7.1 Lymphoma

Extranodal lymphoma can arise in tissues making up Waldeyer's ring as well as in focal aggregates of lymphoid tissue found throughout the oral cavity. These are most often of the non-Hodgkin B cell type, and may or may not be associated with lymphadenopathy or systemic symptoms (so-called "B symptoms") such as fever, night sweats, or weight loss. Lesions generally present as painless submucosal oral masses or enlarged adenotonsillar tissue (Figs. 11.23–11.25). Treatment depends on histologic grading and clinical staging of the tumor, and may involve chemotherapy and/or radiation therapy.

A rare form of Natural Killer/T cell lymphoma, formerly known as *midline lethal granuloma*, can affect the midline hard palate. These lesions are typically very aggressive, with bone and vascular invasion resulting in extensive necrosis and destruction of the palate and nasal tissues. The differential diagnosis for a midline destructive process includes trauma, toxic exposure, infection, and inflammatory disorders. Biopsy is needed for definitive diagnosis, with special testing for immunohistochemical markers. This neoplasm can be very difficult to treat and has a generally poor prognosis.

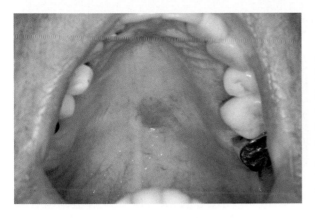

Fig. 11.23 Non-Hodgkin lymphoma of the palate with swelling and erythema.

11.7.2 Leukemias

Overgrowth of malignant hematopoietic cells in the bone marrow with subsequent spillage into the peripheral blood leads to a reduction in the number of normal circulating blood cells. Patients can present with symptoms related to anemia, neutropenia, and thrombocytopenia. Oral findings may consist of gingival bleeding, petechiae, and mucosal ulcers (Fig. 11.26). Oral infections often present atypically, for example dental abscesses may present as soft tissue necrosis without swelling, and recrudescent HSV may present with widespread lesions affecting both the keratinized and nonkeratinized mucosa (Figs. 11.27 and 11.28). Infiltration of malignant cells into the tissues can result in mucosal

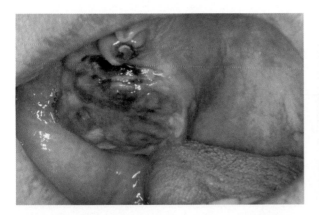

Fig. 11.24 Large right maxillary swelling with ulceration. Incisional biopsy confirmed localized recurrence of previously treated non-Hodgkin lymphoma.

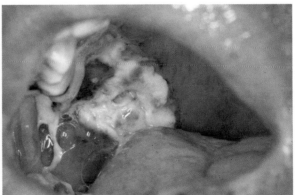

Fig. 11.26 Large neutropenic ulcer of the palate developing in relation to a carious molar in a patient with acute leukemia undergoing induction chemotherapy. The circular appearing depression within the ulcer represents the site of a punch biopsy.

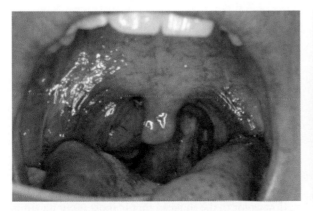

Fig. 11.25 Non-Hodgkin lymphoma of the right palatine tonsil. Note prominent asymmetric enlargement of the right tonsil.

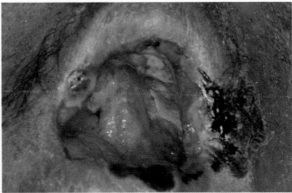

Fig. 11.27 Fulminant recrudescent herpes simplex virus infection in a patient with refractory leukemia.

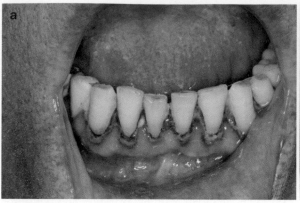

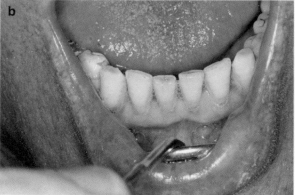

Fig. 11.28 Exacerbation of periodontal disease in a patient with acute leukemia. (**a**) Severe gingival erythema and marginal ulceration in response to heavy calculus deposits on the anterior mandibular teeth. (**b**) Complete resolution of lesions 1 week later following treatment with dental scaling and twice daily chlor-hexidine rinses. Reprinted from Oral Surgery Oral Medicine Oral Pathology Oral Radiology and Endodontology, Vol. 107, Mawardi H, Cutler C, Treister N, *Medical management update: Non-Hodgkin lymphoma*, Pages e19–e33, Copyright (2009), with permission from Elsevier.

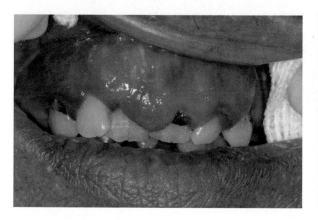

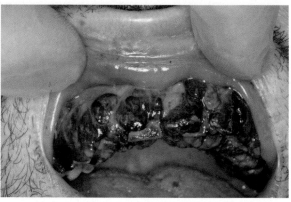

Fig. 11.29 Patient with acute myelogenous leukemia exhibiting prominent gingival involvement. Note sheet-like overgrowth, severe erythema, and focal areas of bleeding.

Fig. 11.30 Severe gingival overgrowth with spontaneous bleeding and areas of focal necrosis in a patient with recently diagnosed myeloproliferative disease.

nodules and gingival enlargement (Figs. 11.29 and 11.30).

11.8 Cowden Syndrome

This is an uncommon autosomal dominant disorder involving hamartomatous growths in multiple organ systems. Raised, nodular lesions can be seen on the lips, face, and intraoral mucosa, often giving tissues a "cobblestoned" or pebbly appearance (Fig. 11.31). The tongue may be prominently fissured. Mucocutaneous lesions are usually benign; however, lesions elsewhere, particularly of the breast and thyroid, have potential for malignant transformation and must be monitored closely.

11.9 Jaundice

Jaundice, occurring secondary to liver disease, bile duct obstruction, and hemolytic disease, can be seen in the oral cavity. Tissue deposition of bilirubin, which is a byproduct of red blood cell breakdown, imparts a yellow color to the mucosa that is most pronounced in the soft palate and floor of mouth (Fig. 11.32).

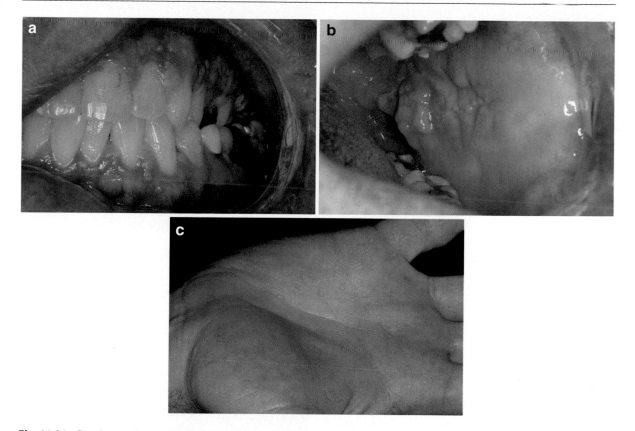

Fig. 11.31 Cowden syndrome. (**a**) Pink, papillary gingival lesions throughout the oral cavity. (**b**) Painless exophytic mass in the posterior buccal mucosa with focal areas of heavy keratinization. (**c**) Multiple painless papules of the palms.

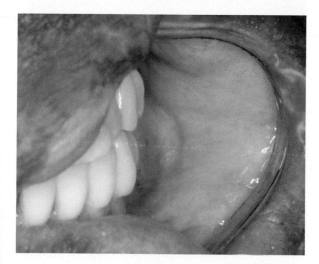

Fig. 11.32 Prominent yellow discoloration of the buccal mucosa in a patient with severe hepatic chronic graft-versus-host disease.

Diagnostic tests: Work-up underlying cause of jaundice.
Biopsy: No.
Treatment: Treatment of underlying medical issue.
Follow-up: Medical follow-up.

11.10   Bisphosphonate-Associated Osteonecrosis of the Jaws

Bisphosphonate-associated osteonecrosis of the jaws (BONJ) is a recently recognized clinical entity that is characterized by exposed nonvital bone in the mandible or maxilla in patients treated with bisphosphonates. Other bones in the body are not affected. Although the vast majority of cases occur in cancer patients treated with high-dose intravenous formulations (primarily for multiple myeloma and metastatic breast, lung, and prostate cancers), there have also been reports of this occurring in patients taking oral preparations for osteoporosis.

Precipitating factors are thought to include oral infections, dental extractions, and local trauma; however, many cases develop spontaneously with no obvious inciting event. Although the precise pathophysiology is unclear, it is likely due to a combination of the following factors: (a) increased bisphosphonate uptake in the jaws relative to long bones, resulting in osteoclast inhibition and profound suppression of bone turnover and repair mechanisms, (b) separation of the oral microflora from the periosteum by only a very thin layer of mucosa that is easily breached, (c) relative frequency of dental infection in the adult population, and (d) routine exposure of alveolar bone during oral surgical procedures.

Lesions appear as yellow or white areas of exposed necrotic bone ranging from a few millimeters to several centimeters in length (Fig. 11.33). The surface may be rough, causing tongue irritation and occasionally traumatic ulceration (Fig. 11.34). The surrounding soft tissue is often erythematous and swollen in response to heavy bacterial colonization of the nonvital bone, and purulent discharge may be noted. Rarely, extraoral fistula formation may develop secondary to deep infection into the bone (Fig. 11.35), or the mandible may become severely brittle and fracture easily (*pathologic fracture*). Although radiographic studies are not required for diagnosis, panoramic radiography or CT imaging should be obtained if the

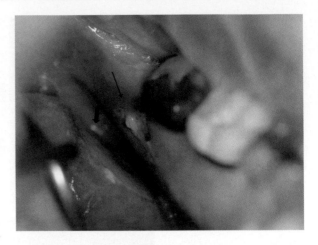

Fig. 11.34 Ulceration of left lateral tongue (*short arrow*) secondary to friction against sharp edges of exposed necrotic bone on the left mylohyoid ridge (*long arrow*). The patient experienced pain radiating down the throat. The bone was smoothed with a file and the ulcer was injected with triamcinolone acetonide, resulting in immediate pain relief and rapid healing. Reprinted from Oral Surgery Oral Medicine Oral Pathology Oral Radiology and Endodontology, Vol. 105, Treister NS, Richardson P, Schlossman R, et al., *Painful tongue ulcerations in patients with bisphosphonate-associated osteonecrosis of the jaws*, Pages e1–e4, Copyright (2008), with permission from Elsevier.

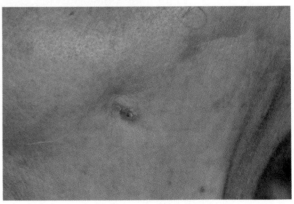

Fig. 11.35 Extraoral fistula in a patient with advanced BONJ of the right mandible.

response to initial therapy is inadequate or complications are suspected (Fig. 11.36).

Treatment is directed at alleviation of symptoms rather than achieving complete wound healing. Sharp bone edges can be smoothed with a small file without the need for local anesthesia, as the bone is nonvital. Mobile bone fragments, or *sequestra*, can likewise be removed with a curette or rongeur (Fig. 11.37). Pain in most cases results from secondary soft tissue infection, which can be treated with topical and/or systemic antimicrobial agents. In cases of recurrent soft

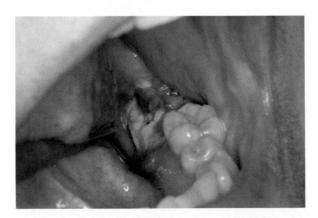

Fig. 11.33 Bisphosphonate-associtated osteonecrosis of the jaw (BONJ) affecting the posterior left mandible following dental extraction. Note ragged appearing necrotic bone and secondarily infected hyperplastic and edematous surrounding soft tissue.

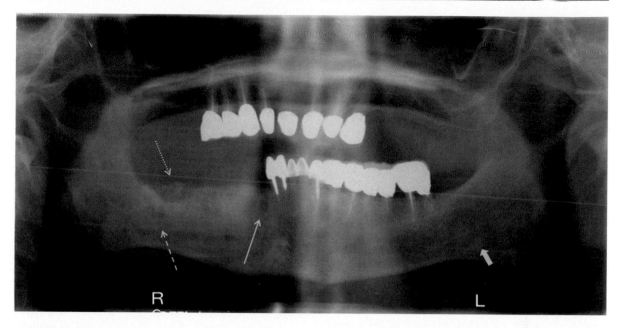

Fig. 11.36 Characteristic radiographic features of BONJ. On the right side, there is a *persistent socket* in the premolar region where a tooth was extracted 2 years previously (*long solid arrow*), *surface irregularity* with bone *sequestration* (*dotted arrow*), and generalized *sclerosis* with loss of definition of the inferior alveolar canal (*dashed arrow*). Note comparison to the left side, which appears relatively normal. The left inferior alveolar canal is clearly visualized (*short solid arrow*).

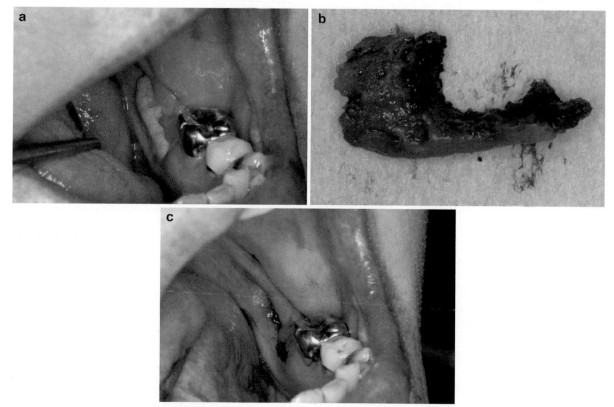

Fig. 11.37 BONJ with a large area of exposed necrotic bone on the left mylohyoid ridge with healthy appearing surrounding soft tissue. (**a**) Palpation of the bone demonstrated slight mobility, indicating a large necrotic bone sequestrum. (**b**) Bony sequestrum that was removed painlessly with a rongeur without local anesthesia. (**c**) Immediately following sequestrum removal.

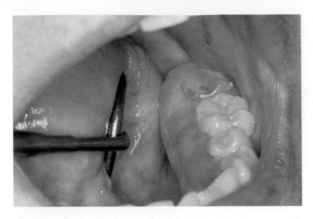

Fig. 11.38 Placement of a protective acrylic stent over the extraction site in the patient from Fig. 11.33 to prevent food impaction and soft tissue irritation.

tissue infection or gross purulence, patients may require long-term systemic therapy. Aggressive surgical intervention should be avoided in the majority of patients. If pain persists with eating despite conservative therapy, fabrication of a surgical stent can be effective in reducing or eliminating symptoms (Fig. 11.38).

Diagnostic tests: None. Consider panoramic radiography or CT if fracture or large sequestrum is suspected.

Biopsy: No, unless there is clinical suspicion for metastatic disease.

Treatment: Only symptomatic lesions require treatment. Rough or irregular bone edges causing tissue irritation should be made smooth and loose nonvital bone fragments should be removed. Soft tissue infection without significant swelling or purulence can typically be managed with chlorhexidine rinses alone; otherwise a 7–10-day course of systemic antibiotic should be prescribed. Ideally, antibiotic selection should be culture directed; however, most organisms are sensitive to the penicillin group. Quinolones, metronidazole, clindamycin, and erythromycin are acceptable alternatives in penicillin-allergic patients. Long-term antibiotic management may be necessary in refractory situations, in particular those with recurrent episodes of pain and swelling.

Follow-up: Patients must be followed closely initially to assess the response to therapy. Patients with stable lesions that are asymptomatic should be reevaluated every 6 months.

Sources

Advisory Task Force on Bisphosphonate-Related Osteonecrosis of the Jaws. American Association of Oral and Maxillofacial Surgeons position paper on bisphosphonate-related osteonecrosis of the jaws. J Oral Maxillofacial Surg 2007;65:369–76

Atmatzidis K, Papaziogas B, Pavlidis T, et al. Plummer-Vinson syndrome. Dis Esophagus 2003;16:154–7

Baccaglini L, Atkinson JC, Patton LL, et al. Management of oral lesions in HIV-positive patients. Oral Surg Oral Med Oral Pathol Oral Radiol Endod 2007;103:S50.e1–23

Badolato R, Fontana S, et al. Congenital neutropenia: advances in diagnosis and treatment. Curr Opin Allergy Clin Immunol 2004;4:513–21

Borges A, Fink J, Villablanca P, et al. Midline destructive lesions of the sinonasal tract: simplified terminology based on histopathologic criteria. AJNR Am J Neuroradiol 2000;21:331–6

Fatahzadeh M, Rinaggio J. Diagnosis of systemic sarcoidosis prompted by orofacial manifestations: a review of the literature. J Am Dent Assoc 2006;137:54–60

Imanguli MM, Pavletic SZ, Guadagnini JP, et al. Chronic graft versus host disease of oral mucosa: review of available therapies. Oral Surg Oral Med Oral Pathol Oral Radiol Endod 2006;101:175–83

Karlinger K, Gyorke T, Mako E, et al. The epidemiology and the pathogenesis of inflammatory bowel disease. Eur J Radiol 2000;35:154–67

Lourenco SV, de Carvalho FR, Boggio P, et al. Lupus erythematosus: clinical and histopathological study of oral manifestations and immunohistochemical profile of the inflammatory infiltrate. J Cutan Pathol 2007;34:558–64

Lu SY, Wu HC. Initial diagnosis of anemia from sore mouth and improved classification of anemias by MCV and RDW in 30 patients. Oral Surg Oral Med Oral Pathol Oral Radiol Endod 2004;98:679–85

Matucci-Cerinic M, Steen VD, Furst DE, et al. Clinical trials in systemic sclerosis: lessons learned and outcomes. Arthritis Res Ther 2007;9 Suppl 2:S7

Ojha J, Cohen DM, Islam NM. Gingival involvement in Crohn disease. J Am Dent Assoc 2008;138:1574–81

Orteu CH, Buchanan JA, Hutchson I, et al. Systemic lupus erythematosus presenting with oral mucosal lesions: easily missed? Br J Dermatol 2001;144:1219–23

Pittock S, Drumm B, Fleming P, et al. The oral cavity in Crohn's disease. J Pediatr 2001;138:767–71

Poate TW, Mouasim KA, Escudier MP, et al. Orofacial presentations of sarcoidosis – a case review and review of the literature. Br Dent J 2008;205:437–42

Rahman A, Isenberg DA. Systemic lupus erythematosus. N Engl J Med 2008;358:929–39

Rodrigo JP, Suarez C, Rinaldo A, et al. Idiopathic midline destructive disease: fact or fiction. Oral Oncol 2005;41:340–8

Scheper MA, Nikitakis NG, Sarlani E, et al. Cowden syndrome: report of a case with immunohistochemical analysis and review of the literature. Oral Surg Oral Med Oral Pathol Oral Radiol Endod 2006;101:625–31

Stewart C, Cohen D, Bhattachraryya I, et al. Oral manifestations of Wegerner's granulomatosis. J Am Dent Assoc 2007;138:338–48

Treister NS, Cook EF, Antin J, et al. Clinical evaluation of oral chronic graft-versus-host disease. Biol Blood Marrow Transplant 2008;14:110–15

Treister N, Sheehy N, Bae EH, et al. Dental panoramic radiographic evaluation in bisphosphonate-associated osteonecrosis of the jaws. Oral Dis 2009;15:88–92

Tomlinson IPM, Houlston RS. Peut-Jeghers syndrome. J Med Genet 1997;34:1007–11

Wijn MA, Keller JJ, Giardiello FM, et al. Oral and maxillofacial manifestations of familial adenomatous polyposis. Oral Dis 2007;13:360–5

Chapter 12
Prescribing Guidelines for Commonly Used Medications

Summary A wide range of topical and systemic medications are used in the management of oral medicine conditions. The vast majority of these therapies are not FDA approved for the specific conditions discussed in this book and are therefore considered "off-label" indications. This chapter provides very specific prescribing guidelines and considerations to ensure that the included medications are used in an appropriate and effective manner for the management of oral diseases.

Keywords Food and drug administration • Cream • Ointment • Gel • Solutions • Candidiasis • Fluconazole • Clotrimazole • Nystatin • Fluocinonide • Clobetasol propionate • Dexamathastone • Tacrolimus • Prednisone • Methylprednisolone • Azathioprine • Colchicine • Dapsone • Hydroxychloroquine • Mycophenolate mofetil • Pentoxyfilline • Thalidomide • Penicillin • Clindamycin • Metronidazole • Amoxicillin/clavulanic acid • Chlorhexidine gluconate • Acyclovir • Valacyclovir • Pilocarpine • Cevimeline • Fluoride • Ibuprofen • Ketoprofen • Clonazepam • Gabapentin • Carbamezapine • Amitriptyline • Nortriptyline • Magic mouthwash • Morphine

Please note that most of the medications included in this book are used "off label" and are therefore not approved by the US Food and Drug Administration (FDA) for the specific clinical indications that are discussed. The information below is meant to be used as a guide and should not replace review of more comprehensive resources such as the Physicians' Desk Reference.

12.1 Inflammatory Conditions

12.1.1 Topical Immunomodulatory Agents

Please note that the package insert for all topical medications will explicitly state that they are "not for use in the oral cavity." While most are not FDA approved for this indication, the medications included in this book are widely used in the practice of oral medicine. It may be helpful to inform both the patient and the pharmacy to avoid any confusion or delays in filling the prescription. *Gels* are preferable to *creams* or *ointments* as they are the most hydrophilic and therefore better absorbed by the wet mucosa. The affected area should be dried with gauze prior to application. The topical agent can be directly applied or mixed with equal parts of a mucoadhesive agent such as Orabase (Colgate-Palmolive, New York, NY) for improved soft tissue retention. Patients should be instructed not to eat or drink for 15–20 min afterward. Alternatively, the topical agent can be applied to gauze placed against the affected tissue for 10–15 min. For lesions restricted to the gingiva and alveolar mucosa, a custom fabricated tray can be used to contain the medication and treat the affected tissues in an intensive manner. Trays should be worn for 15–20 min. Solutions are useful for achieving more widespread topical therapy, and should be swished in the mouth for 5 min then spit out.

In general, topical agents should be applied anywhere from one to six times per day. Any condition requiring more frequent dosing for adequate symptom

J.M. Bruch and N.S. Treister, *Clinical Oral Medicine and Pathology,*
DOI 10.1007/978-1-60327-520-0_12, © Humana Press, a part of Springer Science+Business Media, LLC 2010

control would likely benefit from initiation of systemic treatment in addition to topical therapy.

Secondary candidiasis related to topical corticosteroid therapy is rare but may occur in patients who are predisposed, such as diabetics. If this develops, patients can be treated with topical or systemic antifungal therapy (see Chap. 7). In most cases, subsequent prophylactic treatment with fluconazole 100 mg once or twice weekly is sufficient to prevent recurrence.

- *Fluocinonide gel 0.05%*. Dispense 60 g tube. Dry affected area with gauze and apply with finger. Systemic absorption is generally negligible but has been reported to cause adrenal suppression following prolonged therapy. This is a Class II (high potency) topical corticosteroid.
- *Clobetasol prorpionate gel 0.05%*. Instructions are the same as for fluocinonide gel. This is a Class I (very high potency) topical corticosteroid.
- *Dexamethasone solution 0.1 mg/mL*. Dispense 500 mL for 1 month supply. Swish with 3–5 mL for 5 min then spit. This is the most commonly used topical corticosteroid for oral inflammatory conditions that is commercially available as a solution. Others, such as prednisolone, may also be considered.
- *Tacrolimus 0.1% ointment*. Dispense 60 g tube. Instructions are the same as for topical corticosteroids. Systemic absorption is negligible but has been reported. Topical tacrolimus is only available commercially as an ointment and can be particularly difficult to apply intraorally. Topical tacrolimus has a FDA "black box" warning indicating that its use may be associated with an increased risk of cancer based on animal studies and isolated case reports. This should be discussed with the patient in advance to avoid any confusion or concern when they encounter the warning on the label.
- *Tacrolimus solution 0.1 mg/mL*. This prescription must be prepared by a compounding pharmacist. Dispensing and dosing instructions are the same as for dexamethasone solution. Tacrolimus and dexamethasone can be combined in equal parts of 2 mL each into a single rinse for patients using both agents concurrently.

12.1.2 Systemic Immunomodulatory Agents

- *Prednisone 1 mg/kg* orally as a single morning dose, for 1–2 weeks, for severe immune-mediated ulcerative conditions. Monitor for secondary candidiasis. Begin topical corticosteroid and/or steroid sparing therapy at the same time. The main side effects with short-term therapy include euphoria, insomnia, increased appetite, uncontrolled blood glucose in diabetics, and elevated blood pressure. For limited courses of up to 2 weeks, there is generally no need to taper the dose. For longer treatment periods, the dose should be tapered by 5–10 mg every 1–2 days; there is no "standard" tapering protocol. Patients requiring long-term therapy, even at low doses (e.g. 10 mg), must be followed carefully by their primary care physician for prevention and management of steroid-related complications, such as osteoporosis, diabetes mellitus, avascular bone necrosis, and adrenal insufficiency.
- *Methylprednisolone 4 mg "dose pack."* This is a convenient way to prescribe a short course of corticosteroids for management of acute inflammation, such as intense temporomandibular joint pain. The package comes with 21 tablets and very clear dosing instructions for rapid taper over 6 days. *This prescription is generally inadequate for management of severe oral mucosal disease.*
- *Azathioprine 0.5–1.0 mg/kg/day*. The most common side effects include gastritis, nausea, and vomiting, which can be minimized by taking with food and/or in divided doses. A serious side effect is myelosuppression; therefore, CBC and platelet count should be checked weekly during the first month, twice monthly during the second and third months, and monthly thereafter. Patients with thiopurine *S*-methyl transferase deficiency have an increased risk of myelotoxicity; however, the utility of screening for this condition is unclear. Liver function tests should be checked every 2 weeks during the first month and monthly thereafter.
- *Colchicine 0.6 mg* tablets once or twice daily. Begin once daily and monitor for response for 1–2 weeks before increasing the dose. Common side effects include diarrhea, nausea, and vomiting. CBC should be checked monthly for myelosuppression.
- *Dapsone 50–100 mg* once daily. Patients with glucose-6-phosphate dehydrogenase (G6PD) deficiency, methemoglobin reductase deficiency, or hemoglobin M are at risk for hemolysis. CBC should be monitored weekly for the first month, monthly for the next 6 months, then semiannually. Liver function tests should be drawn at baseline; periodically thereafter if abnormal.

- *Hydroxychloroquine 200–400 mg* once daily with food. Common side effects include diarrhea, nausea, vomiting, myopathy, and headache. CBC should be checked periodically during prolonged therapy. Patients with G6PD deficiency are at risk for hemolysis. Patients on long-term therapy are at risk for irreversible retinopathy and should see an ophthalmologist for a baseline exam and every 3 months thereafter.
- *Mycophenolate mofetil 500 mg* twice daily (1.0 g total daily dose); can increase to 1,000 mg twice daily (2.0 g total daily dose). Medication should be taken on an empty stomach. CBC should be checked weekly during the first month, twice monthly for the second and third months, then monthly through the first year. Renal, hepatic, cardiac, and pulmonary function as well as electrolyte panel should be evaluated periodically.
- *Pentoxyfilline 400 mg* three times daily. Can increase to 800 mg three times daily. Side effects may include nausea, vomiting, dizziness, and headache. Evidence of positive response to medication may take weeks.
- *Thalidomide 50–200 mg* once daily, at night at least 1 h after dinner. The minimum effective dose should be used. Common side effects include edema, rash, hypocalcemia, constipation, nausea, leukopenia, sedation, and peripheral neuropathy. Thalidomide must be discontinued if peripheral neuropathy develops. This medication is only available under a special restricted distribution system call the S.T.E.P.S. Program (System for Thalidomide Education and Prescribing Safety) and prescribing doctors and their patients must be registered.

12.2 Infectious Conditions

12.2.1 Antibacterial Agents

- *Penicillin 500 mg* four times daily for 7–14 days. Take on an empty stomach 1 h before, or 2 h after meals.
- *Clindamycin 150–300 mg* three to four times daily for 7–14 days. This is a good alternative antibiotic for penicillin-allergic patients. The risk of developing secondary pseudomembranous colitis following short-term therapy is now considered to be negligible.

- *Amoxicillin/clavulanic acid 500/125 or 875/125 mg* twice daily for 7–14 days. When used long-term for bisphosphonate osteonecrosis and recurrent soft tissue infection, a single daily dose is typically sufficient. This should be taken with meals.
- *Metronidazole 250 mg* once or twice daily for 7–14 days. Patients should be instructed not to consume alcohol while taking this medication due to a potential disulfiram-like reaction.
- *Chlorhexidine gluoconate 0.12% mouthwash.* Rinse with 5.0 mL twice daily for 30–60 s and spit. This may cause burning in patients with inflammatory mucosal disease. It can also cause dark staining of the teeth that is removable by professional dental cleaning.

12.2.2 Antiviral Agents

- *Acyclovir 400 mg.* For primary herpes infection: 400 mg three times daily for 7–10 days. For episodic reactivation: 400 mg three times a day or 800 mg twice daily for 5 days beginning at the earliest indication of reactivation. For suppressive therapy: 400 mg twice daily. The medication is available in suspension form. Side effects are rare and may include abdominal pain and nausea, headache, and rash.
- *Valacyclovir 500 mg.* This has better bioavailability than acyclovir and requires less frequent dosing. For primary herpes infection: 1.0 g twice daily for 7–10 days. For episodic outbreak: 1–2 g twice daily for 5 days beginning at the earliest sign or symptom. For suppressive therapy: 500 mg once daily.

12.2.3 Antifungal Agents

- *Nystatin suspension 100,000 U/mL.* Swish 5.0 mL for 2–3 min then swallow; four times daily for 1 week. Can be used once daily for prophylaxis.
- *Clotrimazole troches.* Let troche dissolve slowly in the mouth 4–5 times daily for 1 week; one troche daily for prophylaxis. This should not be prescribed in patients with significant salivary gland hypofunction as the troches will not dissolve.
- *Nystatin and triamcinolone cream.* Apply to the corners of the mouth twice daily until angular cheilitis resolves; resume therapy as needed.

- *Fluconazole 100 mg* once daily for 7–14 days depending on extent and severity of candidiasis. For patients on long-term prophylaxis, 100 mg once or twice weekly is generally effective in preventing recurrence. Side effects are rare but may include nausea, vomiting, and increased liver enzyme levels.

12.3   Salivary Gland Hypofunction

12.3.1   *Sialogogues*

- *Pilocarpine 5 mg* three times daily. This can be increased to 10 mg three times daily but side effects are often poorly tolerated. Common side effects include skin flushing, sweating, nausea, and dizziness. This is contraindicated in patients with narrow-angle glaucoma and poorly controlled asthma, and should generally be avoided in patients with chronic obstructive pulmonary disease.
- *Cevimeline 30 mg* three times daily. Instructions are the same as for pilocarpine. This is thought to have slightly more specific affinity for the salivary gland muscarinic receptors.

12.3.2   *Fluoride*

- *Sodium fluoride 1.1% gel*, applied with a toothbrush before bed. The patient should be instructed to expectorate but not rinse with water afterwards. Alternatively, this can be applied in a soft custom tray and left in place for at least 15 min or overnight. A prescription is required.

12.4   Pain Conditions

12.4.1   *Nonsteroidal Antiinflammatory Agents*

- *Ibuprofen 200–400 mg*, every 4–6 h, not to exceed 3,200 mg/day. Common side effects include abdominal pain, nausea, diarrhea, vomiting, rash, increased

liver function tests, and renal failure. This should be used with caution and with dosing adjustment in patients with impaired renal function.

- *Ketoprofen cream 20%. This prescription must be prepared by a compounding pharmacist.* Apply to the skin of the affected area one to four times daily. Side effects from topical therapy are very rare.

12.4.2   *Anticonvulsants*

- *Clonazepam 0.5–1.0 mg* before bed. Patients may note sedation for the first several days but generally develop tolerance to this anticipated side effect. If symptoms recur midday, an additional daytime dose (0.25–0.5 mg) can be considered. Side effects include dizziness, impaired cognition, and sedation. Alcohol should be avoided as clonazepam may potentiate the sedative effects of other CNS depressants as well as prolong metabolism of other drugs that undergo hepatic clearance. Prescribe with caution in patients with a history of substance dependency, as use of benzodiazepines can be habit forming.
- *Clonazepam 1.0 mg tablet topical therapy.* Let the tablet dissolve fully in the mouth (without swallowing saliva) over a 5-min period then spit out. Systemic absorption and associated side effects are negligible.
- *Clonazepam solution 0.1 mg/mL. This prescription must be prepared by a compounding pharmacist.* Swish with 3–5 mL for 5 min then spit, one to three times daily. Dispense appropriate volume based on dosing frequency.
- *Gabapentin 300 mg*: take 300 mg on day 1, 300 mg twice daily on day 2 (600 mg total dose), and 300 mg three times daily on day 3 (900 mg total dose) with maintenance at 900 mg daily thereafter. The total daily dose may be increased up to 1,800 mg in three divided doses if required for symptom control. Common side effects include ataxia, dizziness, sedation, fatigue, myalgia, and peripheral edema. *If side effects are noted with the initial 300 mg dose, then decrease to 100 mg on day 1, 200 mg on day 2, and 300 mg on day 3. The dose may then be carefully increased as tolerated.*
- *Carbamazepine 100 mg* twice daily; can increase by 200 mg/day (divided into two doses), not to

exceed a total dose of 1,200 mg/day. The lowest effective dose should be used. Common side effects include confusion, dizziness, sedation, nausea, vomiting, and lightheadedness. Uncommon but serious side effects include bone marrow suppression with pancytopenia and Stevens–Johnson syndrome. CBC, urinalysis, and liver function tests should be ordered at baseline and then periodically during long-term therapy.

12.4.3 Tricyclic Antidepressants

- *Amitriptyline 10–20 mg* at night before bed. Consider starting with 5.0 mg by splitting the tablet and slowly increasing dosage. Desired effects may not be noted for 2–3 weeks. Common side effects include xerostomia, constipation, dizziness, sedation, fatigue, and weight gain. Alcohol should be avoided due to potentiation of CNS sedative effects. This should not be used in conjunction with monoamine oxidase (MAO) inhibitors.

- *Nortriptyline 25 mg* at night before bed; may drop down to 10 mg if the higher dose is not well tolerated. Side effects are the same as with amitryptyline but may be less pronounced.

12.4.4 Topical Analgesics

- *Two percent viscous lidocaine.* Swish with 2–5 mL for 1 min and spit, as needed. Do not swallow. This can be particularly useful just prior to eating.
- *Magic mouthwash,* consisting of equal parts lidocaine, diphenhydramine, and bismuth subsalicylate solutions. Swish with 2–5 mL for 1 min and spit, as needed. A small amount can be swallowed for severe posterior oropharyngeal pain, but this should only be recommended in adults.
- *Morphine oral solution 10 mg/5 mL.* Swish with 2–5 mL for 5 min and spit, as needed. Do not swallow. This is available in higher a concentration (10 mg/mL) but should be prescribed with caution and is generally used as a salvage therapy to reduce the need for higher doses of systemic analgesics.

Index